Abdelkader Bentouati

Febrile neutropenia in adult cancer

Abdelkader Bentouati

Febrile neutropenia in adult cancer

Protocols and optimized management

ScienciaScripts

Imprint

Cover image: www.ingimage.com

This book is a translation from the original published under ISBN 978-620-8-87145-1.

Publisher:
Sciencia Scripts
is a trademark of
Dodo Books Indian Ocean Ltd. and OmniScriptum S.R.L publishing group

120 High Road, East Finchley, London, N2 9ED, United Kingdom
Str. Armeneasca 28/1, office 1, Chisinau MD-2012, Republic of Moldova, Europe
Managing Directors: Ieva Konstantinova, Victoria Ursu
info@omniscriptum.com

Printed at: see last page
ISBN: 978-620-8-87224-3

Contents

Foreword

Febrile neutropenia remains one of the most feared and frequent complications of cancer treatment. For us, as clinicians involved in the day-to-day care of cancer patients, it represents a medical emergency whose rapid and appropriate management is a major determinant of prognosis. Each episode of febrile neutropenia is a race against time, a challenge in which diagnostic rigour and therapeutic relevance are put to the test.

In the course of my practice and my discussions with my colleagues, whether oncologists, haematologists, infectiologists, emergency physicians or young doctors in training, I have noticed a constant need for a comprehensive, practical and up-to-date resource on this subject. Recommendations are evolving, pathogen spectrums are changing, new strategies are emerging, and it is sometimes difficult to navigate through this mass of information to extract the essential information that can be applied at the patient's bedside.

It is this clinical reality, this shared quest to optimise our practices, that motivated the writing of this book, "**Neutropénie Fébrile en Cancérologie Adulte : Protocoles et Prise en Charge Optimisée**". My primary ambition was to create a tool that could serve as a reliable guide, from an understanding of the physiopathological mechanisms to the most concrete decision-making algorithms, including prevention strategies. I wanted it to be aimed at a wide range of healthcare professionals, so that each could find the level of information best suited to his or her own practice and needs.

This book is the result of an in-depth review of the scientific literature, the recommendations of the main international learned societies and accumulated clinical experience. It has been designed to be resolutely practical, with clearly structured chapters, decision-making algorithms, summary tables and "key points" to make it easier to memorise and apply knowledge. Particular attention has been paid to the most critical aspects: initial risk assessment, choice of empirical antibiotic therapy, management of persistent fevers, management of fungal infections, and prevention strategies using growth promoters and prophylaxis.

I sincerely hope that this book will become a useful companion for all those faced with febrile neutropenia. If this book contributes in any small way to improving the management of our patients, to reducing the morbidity and mortality associated with this complication, and to strengthening the confidence of carers in dealing with this emergency, then its most cherished aim will have been achieved.

I would like to express my deep gratitude to all those who, through their teaching, their work or their exchanges, have enriched my thinking and contributed, directly or indirectly, to the realisation of this project. I hope that you will find this handbook a useful resource and a valuable ally in your day-to-day commitment to patient care.

Dr Bentouati Abdelkader

Introduction

Febrile Neutropenia, an Oncological Emergency

Febrile neutropenia (NF) is one of the most frequent and formidable complications in adult oncology and haematology. A direct consequence of the myelotoxicity of chemotherapy, certain targeted therapies or the invasion of bone marrow by the disease, it plunges patients into a state of profound immunodepression, making them extremely vulnerable to potentially lethal infections. The onset of fever in a neutropenic patient should therefore be considered an absolute medical emergency, requiring immediate assessment and therapeutic intervention to prevent an unfavourable outcome [1].

1. Definition and importance of febrile neutropenia (NF)

Neutropenia is defined as a decrease in the absolute number of neutrophils (PNN) in the blood. It is classically graded according to its severity, with severe neutropenia (PNN < 0.5 G/L or < 500/mm^3) and profound neutropenia (PNN < 0.1 G/L or < 100/mm3) being associated with the highest risk of infection [2]. **Febrile neutropenia** is traditionally defined by the coexistence of fever (single oral temperature > *38.3°C* or temperature > 38.0°C maintained for at least one hour) and neutropenia (PNN < 0.5 G/L, or PNN < 1.0 G/L with a predictable drop below 0.5 G/L within 48 hours) [3, 4].

The importance of NF lies in its potential for significant morbidity and mortality. In the absence of prompt antibiotic treatment, an infection in a neutropenic patient can progress to severe sepsis and septic shock within hours. Historically, mortality associated with untreated NF was very high. Thanks to advances in management - including early empirical antibiotic therapy, optimised supportive care, and the use of granulocyte growth factors - this mortality has fallen considerably, but it remains a major concern, particularly in patients identified as being at high risk [1, 5].

2. Impact on the prognosis of cancer patients and on anti-tumour treatments

In addition to the immediate risk to life, the occurrence of febrile neutropenia has major consequences for the cancer patient's course of treatment:

- **Impact on cancer prognosis:** NF can lead to delays in the administration of chemotherapy courses, dose reductions and even premature cessation of anti-cancer treatment. These changes in therapeutic intensity, which are crucial to the efficacy of many protocols, can compromise the chances of response and, ultimately, the patient's oncological prognosis [6].
- **Morbidity and quality of life:** Episodes of NF are often associated with prolonged hospitalisation, the need for sometimes invasive complementary examinations, and significant anxiety for patients and their families.

Symptoms associated with the infection and treatment (fever, chills, intense fatigue, side effects of antibiotics) have a profound impact on quality of life.

- **Costs to the healthcare system**: Hospital management of NF episodes, including diagnostic investigations, broad-spectrum anti-infective treatments, supportive care and management of complications, represents a **considerable economic burden** for healthcare systems [7].

The prevention and optimal management of NF are therefore crucial not only for the immediate safety of the patient, but also to enable cancer treatment to be administered under the best possible conditions of efficacy and tolerance.

3. Evolution of management concepts and strategies

The management of febrile neutropenia has evolved considerably over the last few decades. Initially, the approach was largely uniform, involving systematic hospitalisation and broad-spectrum intravenous antibiotic therapy for all patients. Advances have made it possible to refine and personalise strategies:

- **Risk stratification:** One of the major advances has been the introduction and validation of prognostic scores, such as the MASCC (Multinational Association for Supportive Care in Cancer) score [8]. These tools make it possible to identify subgroups of patients at "low risk" of complications, paving the way for outpatient or short hospital stay management strategies for a selected proportion of patients, often with oral antibiotic therapy [3, 4].
- **Optimisation of Empirical Antibiotic Therapy:** Recommendations concerning the choice of antibiotic molecules, the place of monotherapy versus dual therapy, and the targeted use of glycopeptides have been clarified. These choices are increasingly guided by risk stratification, clinical severity, suspected sources of infection and the local epidemiology of bacterial resistance. The concepts of therapeutic de-escalation, once the pathogen has been identified and its susceptibility known, have become central to limiting selection pressure and side-effects.
- **Active prevention:** The use of granulocyte growth factors (G-CSF) as primary prophylaxis (before the first cycle of high-risk chemotherapy) and secondary prophylaxis (after an episode of NF) has been shown to reduce the incidence, duration and severity of neutropenia [9]. The indications for anti-infective prophylaxis (antibacterial, antifungal, antiviral) have also been better defined for very high-risk populations.
- **Management of specific infections:** A better understanding of the risk of invasive fungal infections and viral infections in immunocompromised patients, coupled with more effective diagnostic tools (e.g. fungal biomarkers, multiplex PCR), has led to improved management of these often

difficult infections.

- **Current and future challenges:** The emergence and increasing spread of multi-resistant bacteria (MRB) and highly antibiotic-resistant bacteria (HAB) represent a major challenge on a global scale. This requires constant adaptation of empirical antibiotic therapy protocols, reinforcement of hygiene and infection control measures, and active research into new therapeutic options.

4. Objectives and structure of the book

Given the complexity and clinical importance of febrile neutropenia, this book, "**Febrile Neutropenia in Adult Oncology: Protocols and Optimised Management**", has been designed to meet the needs of clinicians - oncologists, haematologists, infectious diseases specialists, emergency physicians, general practitioners, interns in training, as well as specialist nurses and pharmacists - faced with this emergency on a daily basis.

We have a number of objectives:

- **To provide a clear understanding of** the pathophysiology of febrile neutropenia and the associated infectious risks.
- **To provide a practical, evidence-based guide** to risk assessment, aetiological diagnosis and patient stratification.
- **To detail empirical antibiotic therapy protocols**, de-escalation and adaptation strategies.
- **Management of complications**, specific infections and special situations.
- **Present primary and secondary prevention strategies** (G-CSF, prophylaxis).
- **Be an up-to-date resource** incorporating the latest international recommendations and advances in research.

To achieve these objectives, the book is structured in several distinct parts:

- **Part 1** will set out the **fundamentals** of febrile neutropenia, covering its pathophysiology, definitions, epidemiology and the essential risk factors to be aware of.
- **Part 2** will focus on the **diagnostic** approach **and initial assessment of** the patient, detailing the clinical approach, essential paraclinical examinations and risk stratification tools.
- **Part 3**, which forms the core of this book, deals comprehensively **with therapeutic management**. It will explore the principles of empirical antibiotic therapy, strategies for adapting therapy, the management of fungal and viral infections, and the management of associated complications.
- **Part 4** will be devoted entirely to strategies for **preventing** febrile

neutropenia, with particular emphasis on the rational use of granulocyte growth factors (G-CSF) and various anti-infective prophylaxes.

- Finally, **Part 5** will look at **special situations** (such as management of elderly patients and haematological malignancies) and look to the **future**, in particular by discussing the impact of bacterial resistance and new avenues of research in this field.

this field.

Practical **appendices**, including summary algorithms, assay tables and other useful resources, will round off the book, making it a useful reference tool for everyday use.

We hope that this structure will make for clear, progressive and didactic reading, providing every healthcare professional with the knowledge and tools needed for optimised and safe management of febrile neutropenia, thereby helping to improve the prognosis and quality of life of cancer patients.

References

1. Klastersky J, de Naurois J, Rolston K, et al. Management of febrile neutropaenia: ESMO Clinical Practice Guidelines. Ann Oncol. 2016;27(suppl 5):v111-v118.

2. National Cancer Institute. Common Terminology Criteria for Adverse Events (CTCAE) v5.0. Published November 27, 2017. Accessed January 15, 2024.

3. Freifeld AG, Bow EJ, Sepkowitz KA, et al. Clinical practice guideline for the use of antimicrobial agents in neutropenic patients with cancer: 2010 update by the Infectious Diseases Society of America. Clin Infect Dis. 2011;52(4):e56-e93.

4. Taplitz RA, Kennedy EB, Bow EJ, et al. Outpatient Management of Febrile Neutropenia in Adults Treated for Malignancy: American Society of Clinical Oncology and Infectious Diseases Society of America Clinical Practice Guideline Update. J Clin Oncol. 2018;36(14):1443-1453.

5. Kuderer NM, Dale DC, Crawford J, Lyman GH. Mortality, morbidity, and cost associated with febrile neutropenia in adult cancer patients. Cancer. 2006;106(10):2258-2266.

6. Lyman GH, Dale DC, Crawford J. Incidence and predictors of low doseintensity in adjuvant breast cancer chemotherapy: a nationwide study of community practices. J Clin Oncol. 2003;21(24):4524-4531.

7. Aapro MS, Bohlius J, Cameron DA, et al. 2010 update of EORTC guidelines for the use of granulocyte-colony stimulating factor to reduce the incidence of chemotherapy-induced febrile neutropenia in adult patients with

lymphoproliferative disorders and solid tumours. Eur J Cancer. 2011;47(1):8-32.
8. Klastersky J, Paesmans M, Rubenstein EB, et al. The Multinational Association for Supportive Care in Cancer risk index: A multinational scoring system for identifying low-risk febrile neutropenic cancer patients. J Clin Oncol. 2000;18(16):3038-3051.
9. Smith TJ, Bohlke K, Lyman GH, et al. Recommendations for the Use of WBC Growth Factors: American Society of Clinical Oncology Clinical Practice Guideline Update. J Clin Oncol. 2015;33(28):3199-3212.

Part 1

Fundamentals of Febrile Neutropenia

Chapter 1: Pathophysiology of Neutropenia and Infectious Risk

Introduction

Febrile neutropenia is a direct consequence of profound impairment of the host's immune defences, mainly due to a reduction in the number of circulating neutrophils (PNN). To fully understand the issues involved in the diagnosis and management of this oncological emergency, it is essential to understand the underlying pathophysiological mechanisms. This chapter provides a reminder of granulopoiesis and the essential role of NPCs, explores the various causes of neutropenia in oncology, details the mechanisms of induced immunosuppression, and examines how alteration of mucosal barriers promotes microbial translocation, leading to a broad spectrum of potential pathogens.

1.1 Reminder of Granulopoiesis and the Role of Neutrophil Polynuclear Cells (NPCs)

- **1.1.1 Granulopoiesis: Production of NPCs**

Neutrophils, or neutrophil granulocytes, are essential leukocytes of innate immunity, produced in the bone marrow from pluripotent haematopoietic stem cells. This process, known as granulopoiesis, is finely regulated by a combination of cytokines and growth factors, the most important of which is Granulocyte ColonyStimulating Factor (G-CSF) [1]. Granulopoiesis comprises several stages of maturation: myeloblast, promyelocyte, myelocyte, metamyelocyte, non-segmented PNN (or "band"), and finally mature segmented PNN, which are released into the bloodstream.

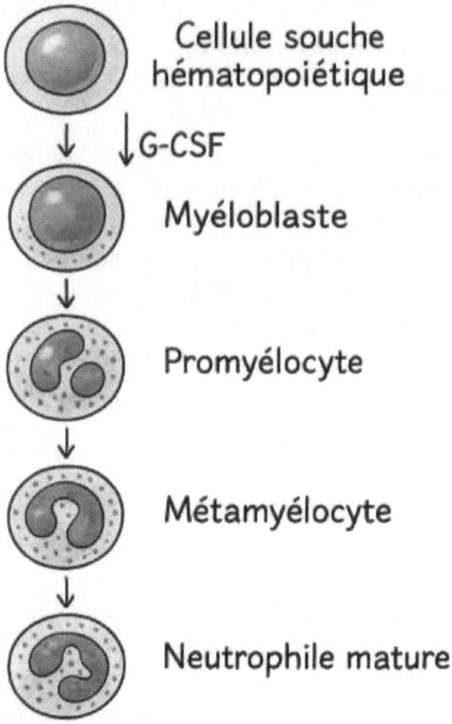

Figure 1.1: Simplified diagram of granulopoiesis. Illustration of the different stages in the maturation of PNN from the haematopoietic stem cell, with mention of the main regulatory factors such as G-CSF.

NPCs have a short half-life in blood (around 6-8 hours) and are produced in very large quantities (around 10¹¹ cells per day in healthy adults) to maintain a circulating pool and a marrow reserve pool [2].

- **1.1.2 Key functions of NPCs in anti-infective defence**

PNN are the first immune cells to be recruited to a site of infection or inflammation. They have multiple crucial functions [2, 3]:

○ **Chemotaxis:** directed migration towards the infectious site in response to chemotactic signals (chemokines, bacterial products, complement fragments).

○ **Phagocytosis:** Recognition, internalisation and destruction of micro-organisms (bacteria, fungi). This process involves surface receptors (e.g. receptors for the Fc fragment of immunoglobulins, complement receptors) and the formation of phagosomes.

○ **Intracellular destruction of pathogens:** Oxygen-dependent (production of reactive oxygen derivatives - ROS - via activation of NADPH oxidase, or "oxidative burst") and oxygen-independent (content of azurophilic and specific granules: lysozyme, elastase, myeloperoxidase, defensins, cathelicidins) mechanisms.

○ **Formation of NETs (Neutrophil Extracellular Traps):** Release of DNA nets and granular proteins that trap and kill extracellular pathogens.

○ **Production of cytokines and chemokines:** Modulation of the inflammatory response and recruitment of other immune cells.

A significant drop in the number of PNN (<0.5 G/L) severely compromises these defence mechanisms, exposing the body to a high risk of serious, disseminated infections.

1.2 Causes of neutropenia in oncology

Neutropenia in cancer patients is most often iatrogenic, but may also be related to the disease itself [4].

- **1.2.1 Myelotoxic chemotherapy :**

This is the most common cause. Many cytotoxic chemotherapy agents target rapidly dividing cells, including haematopoietic precursors in the bone marrow [5].

○ The intensity and duration of neutropenia (the "nadir") depend on the type of chemotherapy (alkylating agents, anthracyclines, taxanes, etc.), the doses used, the administration schedule and individual factors.

○ The nadir generally occurs 7 to 14 days after the administration of chemotherapy.

- **1.2.2 Extensive radiotherapy :**

Irradiation of large volumes of active bone marrow (e.g. pelvic, craniospinal, total body irradiation) can induce significant myelosuppression, including neutropenia [6]. Combination radio-chemotherapy increases this risk.

- **1.2.3 Tumour invasion of the bone marrow :**

Certain haematological malignancies (leukaemia, lymphoma, myeloma) or medullary metastases of solid tumours can infiltrate and destroy the bone marrow, altering normal haematopoiesis [4].

- **1.2.4 Other anti-cancer therapies :**

○ Some targeted therapies may induce neutropenia (e.g. CDK4/6 inhibitors, some tyrosine kinase inhibitors).

○ Immunotherapies (ICIs) may, more rarely, cause immuno-mediated neutropenia (see Chapter 13).

- **1.2.5 Causes not directly related to the treatment or tumour:** ○ Intercurrent viral infections (e.g. CMV, EBV, hepatitis).

○ Vitamin deficiencies (B12, folates) - rare in this context but not to be forgotten.

o Non-oncological drugs (e.g. certain antibiotics, anti-inflammatory drugs, anti-epileptics).
o Hypersplenism (in cases of cirrhosis or portal hypertension).
o Pre-existing autoimmune or haematological diseases.

1.3 Mechanisms of Neutropenia-Induced Immunosuppression

Neutropenia is not limited to a simple quantitative reduction in PNN; it induces a complex state of immunosuppression affecting several components of the immune response [2, 3, 7].

- **Failure of the first line of defence:** loss of the ability to rapidly contain a microbial invasion at the entry sites (mucous membranes, skin).
- **Impaired phagocytosis and pathogen destruction:** Fewer PNN means a reduced capacity to eliminate bacteria and fungi.
- **Impaired signalling and recruitment of other immune cells:** PNNs play a role in initiating and amplifying the inflammatory and adaptive immune response. Their absence disrupts this orchestration.
- **Synergy with other immune deficiencies:**

o Anticancer treatments (chemotherapy, radiotherapy, corticoids) can also induce lymphopenia (affecting T and B lymphocytes), impaired macrophage function, and dendritic cell dysfunction.
o Cancer itself can be a source of immunodepression.
o Nutritional status (frequent malnutrition) and co-morbidities can aggravate immunodeficiency.

This state of global immunodepression, dominated by neutropenia, explains the increased susceptibility to opportunistic infections and the rapidity of their progression.

1.4 Impaired mucosal barriers and risk of bacterial/fungal translocation

Mucosal barriers (digestive, respiratory, oropharyngeal) constitute an essential physical and immunological defence against commensal and pathogenic micro-organisms.

- **Chemotherapy/radiotherapy-induced mucositis:** Many cancer treatments are toxic to rapidly renewing mucosal epithelial cells, causing inflammation, ulceration and disruption of barrier integrity [5, 8].

o Oral and gastrointestinal mucositis is particularly frequent and severe with certain agents (e.g. 5-FU, methotrexate, anthracyclines, ENT or digestive irradiation).

- **Consequences of altered barriers :**

o **Entry point for infections :** Micro-organisms can more easily cross the altered barrier and reach the bloodstream or deep tissues.
o **Microbial translocation:** Passage of commensal bacteria or fungi

(normally contained in the intestinal lumen or on the mucosa) through the damaged intestinal wall or mucosa into the systemic circulation. This is a major mechanism of endogenous infection in neutropenic patients [9].

o Dysbiosis (alteration in the balance of the microbiota) induced by antibiotics or the disease may favour the proliferation of opportunistic pathogens and translocation.

- **Role of intravenous catheters:** Central or peripheral catheters, although necessary, also represent entry points for cutaneous micro-organisms (staphylococci, streptococci, Candida) and can be the site of infectious biofilms.

The combination of neutropenia (lack of systemic defence) and damage to mucosal barriers (facilitating microbial invasion) creates a very high-risk infection situation.

1.5 Spectrum of pathogens involved in febrile neutropenia

The spectrum of micro-organisms responsible for infections in febrile neutropenic patients is broad and has evolved over time [4, 10].

- Bacteria (most frequent) :

o **Gram-negative bacteria (GNB):** Historically predominant and associated with high mortality.

■ Enterobacteriaceae: *Escherichia coli, Klebsiella pneumoniae, Enterobacter spp.* (often resulting from digestive translocation).

■ *Pseudomonas aeruginosa*: Particularly feared for its virulence and resistance.

o **Gram-positive bacteria (GPC):** Their incidence has increased, particularly in connection with the use of central catheters and mucositis.

■ Staphylococci: *Staphylococcus aureus* (including SARM), coagulase-negative staphylococci (SCN, often contaminants but can be pathogenic on catheters).

■ Streptococci: *Streptococcus viridans* (oral translocation, risk of endocarditis), *Streptococcus pneumoniae*, enterococci (including VRE).

o **Anaerobes:** May be involved in polymicrobial infections (abdominal, ENT, skin).

- **Fungi (Invasive Fungal Infections - IFI):**

o Occur especially in cases of profound and prolonged neutropenia (>7- 10 days), use of broad-spectrum antibiotics, or corticosteroid therapy.

o Yeasts: *Candida spp.* (candidaemia, disseminated candidiasis). *Candida albicans* is still common, but non-albicans species are emerging (e.g. *C. glabrata, C. krusei*) which are sometimes resistant to azoles.

o Moulds: *Aspergillus spp* (invasive pulmonary, sinus and disseminated aspergillosis). More rarely, Mucorales (mucormycosis), Fusarium, Scedosporium.

- **Viruses :**

○ Reactivation of latent viruses of the Herpes group: Herpes Simplex Virus (HSV 1 and 2), Varicella-Zoster Virus (VZV), Cytomegalovirus (CMV), Epstein-Barr Virus (EBV).

○ Seasonal respiratory viruses: influenza viruses (Influenza A and B), Respiratory Syncytial Virus (RSV), metapneumovirus, rhinovirus, adenovirus, coronavirus (including SARS-CoV-2).

- **Changes in epidemiological profiles and resistance:**

It is crucial to know the local epidemiology of pathogens and their antibiotic susceptibility profiles (particularly the emergence of multi-resistant BGNs such as ESBL or carbapenemase producers) to guide empirical antibiotic therapy.

Table 1.1: Main pathogens implicated in febrile neutropenia and their frequent routes of entry.

Category of pathogen	Examples of pathogens Keys	Common Entry Points / Sites of Origin
Gram-Negative Negative (BGN)		
	Escherichia coli	Digestive translocation (mucositis), urinary tract infection
	Klebsiella pneumoniae	Digestive translocation, pulmonary infection, urinary tract infection
	Enterobacter spp.	Digestive translocation, catheters
	Pseudomonas aeruginosa	Digestive translocation, water/hospital environment, skin lesions, pulmonary infection, catheters
Gram-positive Bacteria (CGP)		
	Staphylococcus aureus (including MRSA)	Skin, intravenous catheters, oral/nasal mucositis, surgical sites
	Coagulase-negative Staphylococci Negative (SCN)	Skin (commensal flora), intravenous catheters (biofilms)
	Streptococcus viridans group	Translocation from oral mucosa (severe mucositis), oropharynx
	Streptococcus pneumoniae	Upper respiratory tract, lungs
	Enterococci (e.g. *E. faecalis*, *E. faecium*, including VRE)	Digestive tract translocation, urinary tract infection, catheters
Bacteria Anaerobes		
	Bacteroides spp, *Clostridium spp* (e.g. *C. difficile*)	Digestive translocation (mucositis, colitis), polymicrobial infections (abdominal, ENT, soft tissue), abscesses
Fungi (Yeasts)		
	Candida albicans	Digestive translocation (mucositis), intravenous catheters, skin
	Candida spp. non-albicans (e.g. *C. glabrata*, *C. krusei*)	Digestive translocation, intravenous catheters
Fungi (Moulds)		
	Aspergillus spp.	Inhalation of spores (environment), sinuses, lungs
	Mucorales (e.g. *Rhizopus spp.*, *Mucor spp.*)	Inhalation of spores, sinuses, lungs, skin (trauma)
Viruses		
	Herpes Simplex Virus (HSV-1, HSV-2)	Reactivation (oral, genital mucosa), skin
	Varicella-Zoster Virus (VZV)	Reactivation (dermatomes, cutaneous or visceral dissemination)

	Cytomegalovirus (CMV)	Reactivation (lungs, digestive tract, retina)
	Respiratory viruses (Influenza, RSV, Rhinovirus, SARS-CoV-2 etc.)	Respiratory tract (human-to-human transmission, aerosols)

Conclusion

Neutropenia, whether induced by chemotherapy or other cancer-related mechanisms, represents a major failure of the innate immune system. The loss of neutrophils, combined with the frequent alteration of mucosal barriers, exposes patients to a high risk of potentially fulminant infections by a wide range of pathogens. Understanding these pathophysiological mechanisms is the first essential step towards a rational and effective approach to the diagnosis, risk stratification, treatment and prevention of febrile neutropenia, which will be detailed in the following chapters.

References

1. Metcalf D. The granulocyte colony-stimulating factor (G-CSF) family. Oncologist. 2002;7 Suppl 1:16-22.
2. Nathan C. Neutrophils and immunity: challenges and opportunities. Nat Rev Immunol. 2006;6(3):173-182.
3. Mantovani A, Cassatella MA, Costantini C, Jaillon S. Neutrophils in the activation and regulation of innate and adaptive immunity. Nat Rev Immunol. 2011;11(8):519-531.
4. Bodey GP, Buckley M, Sathe YS, Freireich EJ. Quantitative relationships between circulating leukocytes and infection in patients with acute leukemia. Ann Intern Med. 1966;64(2):328-340.
5. Chabner BA, Longo DL. Cancer Chemotherapy and Biotherapy: Principles and Practice. 6th ed. Lippincott Williams & Wilkins; 2018.
6. Yahalom J. Radiotherapy in the era of checkpoint inhibitors: new challenges and opportunities. Leuk Lymphoma. 2018;59(8):1787-1799.
7. Pillay J, den Braber I, Vrisekoop N, et al. In vivo labeling of neutrophils: not so neutral. Blood. 2010;116(1):60-72.
8. Keefe DM, Schubert MM, Elting LS, et al. Updated clinical practice guidelines for the prevention and treatment of mucositis. Cancer. 2007;109(5):820-831.
9. Van Vliet MJ, Tissing WJE, Dun GJ, et al. Chemotherapy-induced gut mucosal damage: an intricate interplay between an Inflamed mucosa, the gut microbiota, and the host immune system. Crit Rev Oncol Hematol. 2020;156:103006.
10. Freifeld AG, Bow EJ, Sepkowitz KA, et al. Clinical practice guideline for the use of antimicrobial agents in neutropenic patients with cancer: 2010 update by the Infectious Diseases Society of America. Clin Infect Dis. 2011;52(4):e56-e93.

Chapter 2: Definitions, Epidemiology and Risk Factors of Febrile Neutropenia

Introduction

Having explored the pathophysiology of neutropenia and associated infectious risk, this chapter focuses on the precise terminology, epidemiological magnitude and determinants of febrile neutropenia (NF). A clear understanding of definitions is essential for consistent communication between healthcare professionals and for the correct application of protocols. By analysing the incidence of NF in different oncology settings and the risk factors that predispose to it, we can identify the most vulnerable populations and guide prevention and management strategies. Finally, we will discuss the factors which, once NF has set in, increase the risk of serious complications or death.

2.1 Precise definitions

Clear, standardised terminology is essential in clinical practice and research.

- 2.1.1 Neutropenia :

Neutropenia is defined by a decrease in the absolute number of circulating neutrophil polynuclear cells (PNN). The most commonly accepted threshold for defining neutropenia is **PNN < 1.5 G/L (or 1500/mm$^{3)}$** . The severity of neutropenia is graded according to the number of PNN, as the risk of infection increases with the depth of neutropenia [1, 2]:

- **Mild neutropenia (CTCAE Grade 1):** PNN 1.0 to < 1.5 G/L.
- **Moderate neutropenia (CTCAE Grade 2):** PNN 0.5 to < 1.0 G/L.
- **Severe neutropenia (CTCAE Grade 3):** PNN < 0.5 G/L (or < 500/mm$^{3)}$. This threshold is often used in the definition of NF. **Agranulocytosis** is also defined as PNN < 0.5 G/L.
- **Profound neutropenia (CTCAE Grade 4):** PNN < 0.1 G/L (or < 100/mm3). Associated with the highest and most serious risk of infection.

The duration of severe neutropenia is also an important prognostic factor (e.g. prolonged neutropenia if > 7-10 days).

Table 2.1: Grades of neutropenia according to CTCAE v5.0.

Grade CTCAE	Description of Neutropenia	Absolute Neutrophil Polynuclear Number (PNN)	Alternative (equivalent) unit	Notes / Common Clinical Implications
Grade 1 Neutropenia	Mild neutropenia	> 1.0 to < 1.5 G/L	> 1000 to < 1500/mm3	Generally low risk of infection.
Grade 2	Moderate neutropenia	> 0.5 to < 1.0 G/L	> 500 to < 1000/mm3	Moderate risk of infection; increased surveillance.
Grade 3	Severe neutropenia	< 0.5 G/L	< 500/mm3	High infectious risk; common threshold for definition of febrile neutropenia (NF).

				Agranulocytosis.
Grade 4	Neutropenia (clinically very profound / life-threatening)¹.	Threshold of < 0.1 G/L often used clinically	< 100/mm3	Maximum infectious risk, often associated with prolonged neutropenia and serious complications.

. 2.1.2 Fever :

In the neutropenic patient, fever is often the first and sometimes the only sign of an underlying infection. The most widely accepted definition of fever in this context is [1, 3] :

○ A **single oral temperature > 38.3°C (101°F)**.

○ OR a **temperature > 38.0°C (100.4°F) maintained for at least one hour**.

It is important to note that some neutropenic patients, particularly those on corticosteroids or the very elderly, may have a serious infection without significant fever. Clinical vigilance is therefore essential, even in the absence of fever, if other signs of infection are present.

- 2.1.3 Febrile neutropenia (NF) :

Febrile neutropenia is therefore defined by the **coexistence of fever (according to the above criteria) AND neutropenia**, most often severe neutropenia [1, 3] :

○ **PNN < 0.5 G/L (or < 500/$mm^{3)}$**.

○ OR **PNN < 1.0 G/L (or < 1000/mm^3)** with a predictable drop below 0.5 G/L in the following 48 hours (e.g. patient at the expected nadir of myelotoxic chemotherapy).

This is the definition adopted by most learned societies and used in clinical trials and management protocols.

2.2 Incidence of Febrile Neutropenia

The incidence of NF varies considerably according to a number of factors, including the type of cancer, the stage of the disease, and above all the type and intensity of anti-cancer treatment administered.

- **2.2.1 Incidence by type of cancer :**

○ **Malignant haemopathies:** The incidence of NF is particularly high in acute leukaemia (up to 80% or more during induction chemotherapy), aggressive lymphomas, and after haematopoietic stem cell transplantation, due to the intensity of treatment and frequent bone marrow involvement [4].

○ **Solid tumours:** The incidence is lower overall but highly variable. It is higher in cancers where chemotherapies are particularly myelotoxic (e.g. breast cancer, small cell lung cancer, sarcomas, germ cell cancers) [5, 6].

- **2.2.2 Incidence according to chemotherapy regimen :**

The risk of NF is directly related to the myelotoxic potential of the chemotherapy regimen used. Learned societies (ASCO, ESMO, NCCN, EORTC) classify chemotherapy regimens according to their risk of inducing NF [1, 7]:

- **High risk (>20% incidence of NF):** e.g. CHOP-21 for lymphoma, TAC for breast cancer, topotecan for ovarian or lung cancer. Primary prophylaxis with G-CSF is generally recommended with these regimens.
- **Intermediate risk (10-20% incidence of NF):** e.g. docetaxel for breast cancer, carboplatin-paclitaxel for ovarian cancer. Primary prophylaxis with G-CSF should be discussed depending on the patient's individual risk factors.
- **Low risk (<10% incidence of NF):** e.g. CMF for breast cancer, monotherapy with 5-FU. Primary prophylaxis with G-CSF is generally not recommended.

Table 2.2: Examples of chemotherapy regimens and their associated risk of febrile neutropenia (NF)
(Source: Adapted from ASCO, ESMO, NCCN, EORTC guidelines [1, 7])

Category of Risk of NF	Incidence of NF	Examples of Chemotherapy	Type of Cancer Frequently Associated	General Recommendation for Primary Prophylaxis with G- CSF
High Risk	> 20%	• CHOP-21 (Cyclophosphamide, Doxorubicin, Vincristine, Prednisone) • R-CHOP-21 • TAC (Docetaxel, Doxorubicin, Cyclophosphamide) • AC-T (Doxorubicin, Cyclophosphamide then Paclitaxel/Dose-dense Docetaxel) • Topotecan (weekly or other high-risk regimen) • Cisplatin + Etoposide (e.g. regimens for CPC) • Induction regimens for Acute Leukaemia	Non-Hodgkin's Lymphoma (NHL) Breast Cancer Breast Cancer Ovarian Cancer, Small Cell Lung Cancer (SCLC) CPC, Germ cell cancers	**Generally recommended**
Risk Intermediate	10-20%	• Docetaxel (monotherapy or certain combinations) • Paclitaxel (weekly) • Carboplatin + Paclitaxel • FOLFIRINOX • Gemcitabine + Cisplatin/Carboplatin • Irinotecan (monotherapy or combinations)	Breast Cancer, Prostate Cancer Breast Cancer, Ovarian Cancer Ovarian Cancer, Non Small Cell Lung Cancer (NSCLC) Pancreatic Cancer, Colorectal Cancer NSCLC, Bladder Cancer Colorectal Cancer	**To be discussed** (depending on the patient's individual risk factors)
Low Risk	< 10%	-CMF (Cyclophosphamide, Methotrexate, 5-Fluorouracil) • 5-Fluorouracil (monotherapy, e.g. colorectal adjuvant) • Capecitabine (monotherapy) • Vinorelbine (monotherapy) • Certain targeted therapies as monotherapy (variable risk profile)	Breast cancer Colorectal cancer Breast Cancer, Colorectal Colorectal Lung cancer, Breast cancer	**Generally not recommended**

The introduction of new targeted therapies or immunotherapies in combination with chemotherapy may also modify these risks.

2.3 Risk Factors for the Occurrence of Febrile Neutropenia

In addition to the type of chemotherapy, many other factors can influence the risk of developing NF. These factors may be related to the patient, the disease or the treatment [1, 5, 6, 7].

- **2.3.1 Patient-related factors :**

o **Age > 65-70 years:** Increased risk due to reduced bone marrow reserves and co-morbidities.

o **Impaired general condition (ECOG PS >2).**

o **Malnutrition, hypoalbuminemia.**

o **Comorbidities:** renal failure, liver failure, diabetes, cardiovascular disease, COPD.

o **History of NF** during a previous cycle of chemotherapy (major risk factor for subsequent cycles).

o **Pre-existing neutropenia** or low PNN count prior to chemotherapy.

o Genetic polymorphisms affecting drug metabolism or bone marrow response (area of research).

- **2.3.2 Factors related to cancer disease :**

o **Type of cancer and advanced stage.**

o **Tumour invasion of bone marrow.**

o Lymphoma or leukaemia.

- **2.3.3 Treatment-related factors :**

o **Type and intensity of chemotherapy** (see section 2.2.2).

o **Concomitant or prior extensive radiotherapy** to active bone marrow sites.

o **Absence of primary G-CSF prophylaxis** where indicated.

o Recent major surgery.

o Use of central venous catheters (may promote infection, but not NF directly).

Identification of these risk factors is essential to assess the individual risk of each patient and decide on the indication for G-CSF prophylaxis with intermediate-risk regimens.

2.4 Risk Factors for Serious Complications or Mortality in Established Febrile Neutropenia

Once a patient develops NF, certain factors are associated with a poorer prognosis, i.e. an increased risk of severe complications (sepsis, septic shock, organ failure) or death. Identification of these factors is at the heart of risk stratification (e.g. MASCC score) to guide treatment decisions (hospitalisation vs outpatient treatment, type of antibiotic therapy) [1, 3, 9].

- **Expected Depth and Duration of Neutropenia :**

o PNN < 0.1 G/L (profound neutropenia).

o Severe neutropenia expected to last > 7-10 days.

- **Signs of Sepsis or Haemodynamic Instability at Initial Presentation:**

o Arterial hypotension (SAP < 90 mmHg).

o Tachycardia, tachypnoea.

o Altered level of consciousness.

o Signs of organ hypoperfusion.

- **Significant comorbidities :**

o Renal insufficiency (high creatinine).

o Liver failure (elevated bilirubin).

o Chronic pulmonary disease (COPD) with respiratory symptoms.

o Congestive heart failure.

o Poorly controlled diabetes.

- **Clinically evident and severe outbreak of infection:**

o Documented pneumonia.

o Proven catheter infection.

o Extensive skin or soft tissue infection.

o Severe mucositis (Grade 3-4).

o Severe colitis or diarrhoea.

- **Other factors :**

o Hospitalisation at time of onset of fever.

o Advanced age (especially if associated with frailty or co-morbidities).

o Patients who have received an allogeneic haematopoietic stem cell transplant.

o History of infection with multi-drug resistant bacteria.

o Failure to control fever rapidly on initial antibiotic therapy.

o Some of these factors are included in the calculation of the MASCC score (see Chapter 5).

Table 2.3: Risk factors for the development of febrile neutropenia (NF)
(Source: Adapted from references [1, 5, 6, 7])

Category	Risk factors	Impact on risk of NF
Patient factors	• Age > 65-70 years	Increased risk, especially in
	• Impaired general condition (ECOG PS >2)	combined with
	• malnutrition/hypoalbuminemia	chemotherapy
	• Comorbidities (myelosuppressive renal/hepatic insufficiency, diabetes, COPD, etc.)	myelosuppressive.
	• History of NF	
	• Pre-existing neutropenia (low PNN)	

	• Genetic polymorphisms (under research)	
Disease-related factors	-Advanced or invasive cancer bone marrow compromised. • Lymphoma/leukaemia • Metastatic tumours (bone marrow)	Higher risk due to compromised bone marrow
Treatment-related factors	• High-risk chemotherapy (ex: anthracycline-containing regimens dense dose taxanes) • Extensive bone marrow radiotherapy • Absence of G-CSF prophylaxis • Recent major surgery • Central venous catheters (indirect infectious risk)	Significant increase if combination of several factors.

Table 2.4: Risk factors for serious complications/mortality in established NF

(Source: MASCC score and guidelines [1, 3, 9])

Category	Risk Factors	Impact on prognosis
Severe neutropenia	• PNN < 0.1 G/L • Expected duration > 7-10 days	Increased risk of sepsis and organ failure.
Clinical signs severe	• Hypotension (PAS < 90 mmHg) • Tachycardia/tachypnoea • Altered consciousness • Hypoperfusion	Life-threatening: requires treatment hospital care intensive care.
Comorbidities	• Renal/hepatic failure • Symptomatic COPD • Poorly controlled diabetes • Heart failure	Worsening prognosis and Reduced response to treatments.
Infectious outbreaks	• Respiratory disease • Catheter infection • Severe mucositis (Grade 3-4) • Severe colitis/diarrhoea	Increased risk of septic shock and mortality.
Other factors	• Initial hospitalisation • Advanced age + frailty • HSC allograft • Multi-resistant bacteria • Persistent fever on antibiotics	Included in the score MASCC to stratify risk (high vs. low).

Recognition of these risk factors for poor prognosis is crucial for aggressive and often hospital-based management of the patients concerned.

Conclusion

Febrile neutropenia is a well-defined clinical entity, the incidence of which is strongly influenced by the type of cancer and the chemotherapy regimen used. Knowing the risk factors for developing NF makes it possible to optimise prevention strategies, particularly through the targeted use of G-CSF. Once NF has occurred, identification of the risk factors for serious complications is essential in order to stratify patients and adapt the intensity of therapeutic management. The following chapters will use these definitions and risk concepts to detail the diagnostic approach and treatment protocols.

References

1. Taplitz RA, Kennedy EB, Bow EJ, et al. Outpatient Management of Febrile Neutropenia in Adults Treated for Malignancy: American Society of Clinical Oncology and Infectious Diseases Society of America Clinical Practice Guideline Update. J Clin Oncol. 2018;36(14):1443-1453.
2. National Cancer Institute. Common Terminology Criteria for Adverse Events (CTCAE) v5.0. Published November 27, 2017. Accessed January 15, 2024.
3. Freifeld AG, Bow EJ, Sepkowitz KA, et al. Clinical practice guideline for the use of antimicrobial agents in neutropenic patients with cancer: 2010 update by the Infectious Diseases Society of America. Clin Infect Dis. 2011;52(4):e56-e93.
4. Viscoli C, Varnier O, Machetti M. Infections in patients with febrile neutropenia: epidemiology, microbiology, and risk stratification. Clin Infect Dis. 2005;40 Suppl 4:S240-S245.
5. Kuderer NM, Dale DC, Crawford J, Lyman GH. Mortality, morbidity, and cost associated with febrile neutropenia in adult cancer patients. Cancer. 2006;106(10):2258-2266.
6. Lyman GH, Kuderer NM, Crawford J, et al. Predicting individual risk for neutropenic complications in patients receiving cancer chemotherapy. Cancer. 2011;117(9):1917-1927.
7. Aapro MS, Bohlius J, Cameron DA, et al. 2010 update of EORTC guidelines for the use of granulocyte-colony stimulating factor to reduce the incidence of chemotherapy-induced febrile neutropenia in adult patients with lymphoproliferative disorders and solid tumours. Eur J Cancer. 2011;47(1):8-32.
8. Klastersky J, Paesmans M, Rubenstein EB, et al. The Multinational Association for Supportive Care in Cancer risk index: A multinational scoring system for identifying low-risk febrile neutropenic cancer patients. J Clin Oncol. 2000;18(16):3038-3051.

Part 2

Diagnosis and Initial Assessment

Chapter 3: Initial Clinical Assessment of the Febrile Neutropenic Patient

Introduction

When a patient undergoing cancer treatment presents with fever and suspected neutropenia, the initial clinical assessment is a crucial and urgent step. It aims to rapidly confirm the diagnosis of febrile neutropenia (NF), identify signs of immediate severity, search for a potential infectious site, and gather the information needed to stratify the patient's risk and guide empirical therapeutic management. A systematic approach, combining a targeted history and a thorough, targeted clinical examination, is essential to ensure that key factors that could influence prognosis are not overlooked. This chapter details the steps involved in this initial clinical assessment.

3.1 Recognising the emergency: Identifying the warning signs

Febrile neutropenia is a medical emergency. The first step is to recognise the situations that require immediate intervention and potentially emergency hospitalisation, even before all the results of complementary examinations have been obtained.

- **Signs of haemodynamic instability or severe sepsis :**

o Arterial hypotension (Systolic Blood Pressure < 90 mmHg or fall > 40 mmHg from baseline).

o Tachycardia (> 100-120/min at rest).

o Tachypnoea (> 22-25/min).

o Marbling, cold extremities, prolonged skin recolouring time (> 3 seconds).

o Altered state of consciousness (confusion, agitation, drowsiness).

o Oliguria (< 0.5 mL/kg/h for at least 2 hours despite fluid resuscitation).

These signs suggest severe sepsis or septic shock and require intensive care or resuscitation if necessary [1, 2].

- **Signs of respiratory distress :**

o Rest dyspnoea, orthopnoea.

o Use of accessory respiratory muscles, draught.

Cyanosis.

Oxygen saturation < 90-92% on room air.

- **Acute neurological signs :**

o Disturbances of consciousness (see above).

o Signs of meningitis (intense headache, neck stiffness, photophobia - although neck stiffness may be absent in neutropenic patients).

o Recent focal neurological deficit.

o Convulsive seizures.

- **Other signs of seriousness :**

o Severe, uncontrollable pain.

Significant active bleeding (if associated with thrombocytopenia).

Grade 3-4 mucositis (extensive ulceration, inability to eat).

o Profuse diarrhoea with signs of dehydration.

The presence of one or more of these warning signs should lead to **immediate treatment, often in hospital**, and rapid initiation of empirical antibiotic therapy after sampling (see Chapter 6).

Table 3.1: Clinical warning signs of febrile neutropenia (NF) requiring urgent management *(Source: Adapted from IDSA/ESMO/ASCO guidelines [1, 2, 3])*.

Category	Clinical Signs	Immediate Action
Instability Hemodynamic / Sepsis	• Hypotension (PAS < 90 mmHg or ¿ > 40 mmHg vs baseline) • Tachycardia (> 120/min) • Tachypnoea (> 25/min) • Marbling/cold extremities • Oliguria (< 0.5 mL/kg/h) • Altered consciousness	• Emergency hospitalisation • IV fluid resuscitation • Empirical antibiotic therapy in < 1 hour • Samples microbiological
Distress Respiratory	- Rest dyspnoea/SatO? < 90% - Cyanosis - Pulling/use of accessory muscles	- Immediate oxygen therapy - Chest X-ray - Assessment for pneumopathy/septic shock
Signs Neurological	- Disturbance of consciousness (confusion, coma) - Meningeal signs (headache + photophobia) - Focal deficit or convulsions	• Urgent brain scan • Lumbar puncture (if stable) • Anti-encephalitis antibiotics
Other serious signs	• Severe uncontrollable pain • Active bleeding (if thrombocytopenia) • Grade 3-4 mucositis • Profuse diarrhoea + dehydration	• Correction of fluid and electrolyte disorders • IV analgesia • Transfusion if necessary

Management of NF with warning signs

1. **Assess ABC** (Airway-Breathing-Circulation) :

o Ensure oxygenation and peripheral venous access.

o Start crystaloids (e.g. 0.9% NaCl) in the event of hypotension.

2. **Rapid sampling** :

o Blood cultures x2 (peripheral + catheter if present).

Biological work-up: CBC, CRP, creatinine, ionogram, lactate.

3. **Empirical antibiotic therapy** :

o In < 1h if sepsis/shock (eg: Piperacillin-Tazobactam 4.5g IV or Cefepime 2g IV).

4. **Hospital admission** :

o Intensive care unit if severe shock/sepsis.

3.2 Targeted and systematic history-taking

A rapid but complete history is essential to guide diagnosis and management.

- **3.2.1 Oncological background and recent treatments :**

o Type of cancer, stage, current or recent anticancer treatments (nature of chemotherapy, date of last cycle - to estimate the expected nadir of neutropenia).

o Recent or current radiotherapy (location, extent).

o Recent surgery.

o Presence of a central venous catheter (type, date of insertion, signs of inflammation at the insertion point).

- **3.2.2 Characteristics of Fever and Associated Symptoms :**

o Date and mode of onset of fever, maximum temperature, chills.

o Search for symptoms pointing to an infectious source:

▪ **ENT/Pulmonary:** Cough, sputum (appearance, colour), dyspnoea, chest pain, rhinorrhoea, odynophagia.

▪ **Digestive:** Abdominal pain, nausea, vomiting, diarrhoea (frequency, consistency, presence of blood or mucus), urinary burning, back pain.

▪ **Cutaneous:** Rash, pruritus, pain or discharge from a wound or puncture site.

▪ **Neurological:** Headache, confusion, visual disturbances.

▪ **Other:** Myalgias, arthralgias.

- **3.2.3 Comorbidities and history :**

o Chronic diseases (cardiac, pulmonary, renal, hepatic, diabetes).

o History of recurrent or specific germ infections (e.g. BMR).

o Drug allergies (particularly to antibiotics).

o Vaccination status.

- **3.2.4 Current prophylaxis and treatment :**

o Granulocyte growth factor (G-CSF) intake: type, date of last injection.

o Current antibiotic, antifungal or antiviral prophylaxis.

o Other drugs (corticosteroids, immunosuppressants, NSAIDs, etc.).

3.2.5 Epidemiological context :

o Recent travel.

o Contact with sick people (relatives, recent hospitalisation).

o Exposure to animals.

o Food (raw, unpasteurised products).

3.3 Complete and directed clinical examination in search of an outbreak of infection

The clinical examination of neutropenic patients must be meticulous, as the classic signs of inflammation may be attenuated or absent due to the PNN deficit. The aim is to identify any infectious sites, which will guide microbiological sampling and sometimes the choice of antibiotic therapy.

- **3.3.1 General examination :**

o Take vital signs: temperature, heart rate, blood pressure (lying down and standing up if possible), respiratory rate, oxygen saturation.

o State of consciousness, state of hydration.

o Weight.

- **3.3.2 Skin examination :**

o Look for rash, erythema, heat, pain, induration, pustules, vesicles, ulcerations, pressure sores.

o Inspection of skin folds (axillary, inguinal, submammary).

o **Careful examination of central and peripheral venous catheter insertion sites:** look for redness, pain, induration, discharge.

Examination of the nails (paronychia).

- **3.3.3 Examination of the ENT and Buccal Spheres :**

o **Oral mucosa:** Look for mucositis (erythema, ulcerations, pseudomembranes), oral candidiasis (thrush), herpetic lesions. Dental condition.

o Oropharynx: appearance of tonsils, presence of posterior discharge.

Palpation of cervical lymph nodes.

o Sinus examination (pain on palpation).

- **3.3.4 Pulmonary examination :**

o Inspection (pulling, use of accessory muscles), palpation, percussion.

Pulmonary auscultation: look for crackles, sibilance, decreased vesicular murmur, pleural friction.

- **3.3.5 Cardiovascular examination :**

o Cardiac auscultation: rhythm, heart murmurs, search for a murmur (endocarditis?), pericardial rub.

Palpation of peripheral pulses.

- **3.3.6 Abdominal examination :**

o Inspection, auscultation (hydro-aeric noises), palpation (look for pain, tenderness, contracture, mass, hepatomegaly, splenomegaly), percussion.

Palpation of the lumbar fossa.

- **3.3.7 Examination of the anal and perineal area :**

o **Crucial and often neglected.** Must be carried out with tact and caution.

Inspection for anal fissure, perianal abscess, perineal cellulitis, herpetic lesions.

Rectal examination is generally **contraindicated** in cases of severe neutropenia because of the risk of bacteremia and damage to the mucosa, unless there is a strong clinical suspicion of a deep abscess.

- **3.3.8 Neurological examination Summary (more detailed if symptoms) :**

o State of consciousness, orientation.

Look for meningeal signs (neck stiffness - may be absent).

o Look for focal signs.

- **3.3.9 Osteoarticular examination :**

o Look for joint or bone pain or inflammatory signs.

3.4 The importance of examining "silent" sites in the neutropenic patient

Because of the attenuated inflammatory response due to neutropenia, clinical signs of infection may be discrete or even absent at certain sites. Particular attention should be paid to these "mute" sites, where infection may develop insidiously:

- **Oral mucosa and oropharynx:** Even apparently minor mucositis can be a gateway to serious infections.
- **Sinuses:** Sinusitis may manifest itself only as clear rhinorrhoea or facial heaviness, without the classic signs of pain or localised fever.
- **Peri-Anal and Perineal region**: Infections in this area (cellulitis, abscesses) may initially be of little symptom but rapidly become extensive and serious. Simple discomfort or pain during defecation should raise the alarm.
- **Catheter insertion sites:** A tunnel or implantable chamber infection may have only minimal local signs (discrete redness or sensitivity).
- **Digestive tract**: Neutropenic enterocolitis (typhlitis) may present as diffuse abdominal pain with no obvious peritoneal signs at first.
- **Lungs:** Incipient pneumonitis may have no auscultatory signs. A chest X-ray should therefore be taken systematically.

The active and repeated search for an infectious site, paying particular attention to these "silent" sites, is a key element in the initial assessment and follow-up of the febrile neutropenic patient.

Conclusion

The initial clinical assessment of a patient suspected of having febrile neutropenia is a critical stage which must be carried out rigorously and promptly. Recognition of warning signs pointing to a life-threatening emergency, a targeted history to contextualise the febrile episode, and a thorough and meticulous clinical examination to look for an infectious site (paying particular attention to "silent" sites) are the cornerstones of this assessment. These clinical elements, combined with the results of the initial paraclinical examinations (detailed in the next chapter), will help to confirm the diagnosis, stratify the patient's risk, and guide the initial therapeutic management, particularly the choice of empirical antibiotic therapy.

References

1. Freifeld AG, Bow EJ, Sepkowitz KA, et al. Clinical practice guideline for the use of antimicrobial agents in neutropenic patients with cancer: 2010 update by the Infectious Diseases Society of America. Clin Infect Dis. 2011;52(4):e56-e93.

2. Dellinger RP, Levy MM, Rhodes A, et al. Surviving Sepsis Campaign: international guidelines for management of severe sepsis and septic shock, 2012. Crit Care Med. 2013;41(2):580-637.

3. Klastersky J, de Naurois J, Rolston K, et al. Management of febrile neutropaenia: ESMO Clinical Practice Guidelines. Ann Oncol. 2016;27(suppl 5):v111-v118.

Chapter 4: Emergency Laboratory Tests in Febrile Neutropenia

Introduction

After the initial clinical assessment of a patient suspected of having febrile neutropenia (NF), rapid and targeted paraclinical investigations are essential. These tests have several aims: to confirm neutropenia, assess the patient's general condition and the presence of organ failure, identify any pathogens responsible for the febrile episode, and look for an infectious site that is not clinically evident. The results of these investigations, coupled with the clinical data, will enable the patient's risk to be stratified and the therapeutic strategy, particularly the empirical antibiotic therapy, to be adapted as best as possible. This chapter describes the initial biological work-up, systematic and targeted microbiological sampling, and first-line imaging.

4.1 Initial biology work-up: Assessing the patient's condition and inflammation

A blood sample should be taken as a matter of urgency, ideally before antibiotic therapy is started (unless this significantly delays its administration in cases of severe sepsis).

- **4.1.1 Blood Count (CBC) - Platelets :**

o **Confirmation and quantification of neutropenia:** Determination of the absolute number of neutrophil polynuclear cells (PNN) to confirm the diagnosis of neutropenia and assess its severity (mild, moderate, severe, profound).

o **Other blood lines:**

▪ Haemoglobin: Search for anaemia (pre-existing, chemotherapy-induced, or haemolytic).

▪ Platelets: Check for thrombocytopenia (common after chemotherapy, may be aggravated by infection or DIC).

▪ Lymphocytes: Severe lymphopenia may increase immunosuppression.

• **4.1.2 Renal and electrolyte tests :**

o **Serum creatinine and blood urea:** To assess basic renal function and look for acute renal failure (ARF), which may be a complication of sepsis or drug-induced nephrotoxicity.

o **Blood ionogram (Na+, K+, Cl-, bicarbonates):** Search for electrolyte disorders (e.g. hypokalaemia, hyponatraemia, metabolic acidosis) related to fever, digestive losses, or AKI.

• **4.1.3 Liver function tests :**

o **Transaminases (ASAT, ALAT), Alkaline phosphatases (PAL), Gamma-Glutamyltransferase (GGT), Bilirubin (total and conjugated) :** To detect possible hepatic cytolysis or cholestasis, which may be infectious (e.g. viral hepatitis, sepsis with hepatic involvement), drug-induced, or related to tumour progression.

- **4.1.4 Inflammation and infection markers :**

◦ **C-Reactive Protein (CRP): A** sensitive marker of inflammation and infection. Its level is generally high in NF of infectious origin. Its kinetics can help to monitor progress under treatment [1].

◦ **Procalcitonin (PCT):**

■ **Why:** PCT is considered a more specific marker of bacterial infection than CRP. Elevated levels (>0.5-2 ng/mL) are consistent with systemic bacterial infection or sepsis [2, 3]. It can help distinguish a fever of bacterial origin from a fever of other origin (viral, fungal, non-infectious inflammatory, paraneoplastic).

■ **Limitations:** Its sensitivity and specificity are not perfect. False positives (trauma, recent surgery, certain tumours, pancreatitis, certain irAEs) and false negatives (localised infections, infections with atypical or intracellular germs, very early onset of infection) are possible. Its measurement should not delay the initiation of antibiotic therapy in cases of strong clinical suspicion. It is particularly useful in combination with clinical data and other markers, and its kinetics can help guide the duration of antibiotic therapy (de-escalation) [3, 4].

Table 4.1: Initial laboratory work-up in febrile neutropenia (NF)
(Source: Adapted from references [1-4])

Parameter	Elements Assayed	Interpretation / Clinical implications	Critical values
Blood count Blood cell count count (CBC)	• Absolute neutrophils (PNN) • Haemoglobin (Hb) • Platelets • Lymphocytes	• **PNN < 500/gL**: severe neutropenia • **PNN < 100/gL**: profound neutropenia (major risk of infection) • Anemia (Hb < 8 g/dL): Transfusion to be assessed • Thrombocytopenia (< 50,000/pL): Bleeding risk	PNN < 500/pL Infectious risk $
Renal work-up	• Serum creatinine • Urea • Lonogram (Na^+, K^+, Cl, bicarbonates)	• **ARF**: creatinine > 1.5x baseline • **Electrolyte disorders** : Hypokalaemia, hyponatraemia, metabolic acidosis (related to sepsis/dehydration)	Creatinine > 2 mg/dL Adjust ATB
Work-up Hepatic	• AST/ALT • PAL/GGT • Bilirubin (total/conjugated)	• **Cytolysis** (ASAT/ALAT f) : Toxidermia, viral hepatitis • **Cholestasis** (PAL/GGT t) : Sepsis, obstruction • Bilirubin > 2x N: Risk of complications	Bilirubin > 5 mg/dL Increased surveillance
Inflammatory markers	**- CRP** **- Procalcitonin (PCT)**	- **CRP > 100 mg/L**: probable bacterial infection - **PCT** : - **< 0.5 ng/mL**: Infection unlikely	PCT > 10 ng/mL Severe sepsis

- **0.5-2 ng/mL**: Possible infection
- **> 2 ng/mL**: probable sepsis

Interpretation of Procalcitonin (PCT) in NF

(Based on [2-4])

PCT level (ng/mL)	Interpretation	Clinical Action
< 0,5	Bacterial infection low probable	Re-evaluate origin of fever (viral, fungal, paraneoplastic)
0,5 - 2	Bacterial infection possible	Maintain TBA if clinical signs signs
>2	Bacterial infection systemic or sepsis likely	Broad-spectrum antibiotics + systemic close monitoring
Kinetics	j PCT within 48-72h: Good response to TBA t PCT: Possible therapeutic failure	Adjust TBA or broaden spectrum

- 4.1.5 Other laboratory tests (depending on the context) :

- **Arterial blood gas:** if signs of respiratory distress, shock or severe sepsis (look for hypoxia, lactic acidosis).

Serum lactates: Marker of tissue hypoperfusion and severity of sepsis.

- **Haemostasis work-up (PT, APTT, fibrinogen, D-dimer):** If there are signs of bleeding or DIC, or before an invasive procedure.
- **Blood glucose:** especially in diabetic patients or those on corticosteroids.

4.2 Systematic and directed microbiological sampling: Identifying the culprit

The aim of microbiological sampling is to identify the pathogen responsible for the febrile episode and to determine its susceptibility to antibiotics, so that targeted treatment can be adapted. These samples should be taken **before empirical antibiotic therapy is started**, wherever possible, but without delaying its administration by more than one hour in the case of high-risk NF or signs of sepsis [1, 5].

- 4.2.1 Blood cultures: the cornerstone of bacterial diagnosis

- **Systematic and urgent** in all febrile neutropenic patients.
- **Procedure: At least two pairs of blood cultures** (one pair = one aerobic and one anaerobic bottle).
  - If the patient has a central venous catheter (CVC): collect **one pair from each lumen of the CVC AND one pair from the peripheral venous line**. This makes it possible to calculate the differential positivity time (DTP) which, if it is > 2 hours in favour of the CVC, is a strong argument for a catheter-related infection (CLI) [6].
  - If no CVC: two pairs taken from two separate peripheral venipuncture sites.
- Volume of blood per vial: 8-10 mL in adults.
- Strict asepsis must be observed during sampling to avoid contamination.

o Blood cultures remain positive in only 10-30% of NF episodes, but their positivity has a major impact on management [5].

- 4.2.2 Urine cytobacteriological examination (UCE):

o **Systematic**, even in the absence of urinary symptoms, as urinary tract infections may be paucisymptomatic in neutropenic patients.

o Collect the second stream of urine after local cleansing, or from a urinary catheter if present (do not collect from the collection bag).

urinary catheter if present (do not collect from the collection bag).

- 4.2.3 Directed sampling according to clinical call points :

o **ENT/Pulmonary :**

▪ Throat swab if sore throat or pharyngitis.

▪ Sputum cytobacteriological examination (ECBC) if productive cough (often difficult to obtain in neutropenic patients).

▪ Nasopharyngeal aspirate or swab for respiratory viruses by PCR (influenza, RSV, SARS-CoV-2, etc.) if respiratory symptoms or epidemic context.

▪ Bronchoalveolar lavage (BAL) by bronchial fibroscopy if pneumopathy has been documented without an aetiological diagnosis (see section 4.3.2).

o **Digestive tract:**

▪ Stool culture if diarrhoea, with specific search for *Clostridioides difficile* toxins.

▪ Search for Norovirus or other enteric pathogens by PCR in stools if gastroenteritis.

o **Skin and Soft Tissue:**

▪ Sampling of a suspected skin lesion (pustule, bulla, ulceration, cellulitis) by swabbing, needle puncture or skin biopsy for direct examination and bacterial and fungal culture.

▪ Catheter port sampling if local inflammatory signs.

▪ Puncture of a collection if present.

o **Cerebrospinal fluid (CSF):**

▪ Lumbar puncture (after brain imaging if focal neurological signs or ICCH) if meningitis or encephalitis suspected (intense headache, stiff neck, confusion, consciousness disorders). Cytological, biochemical, bacteriological (direct examination, culture, PCR) and viral analysis.

o **Other samples:** Puncture of joint effusion if arthritis, ascites, etc.

Table 4.2: Microbiological samples taken in febrile neutropenia (NF) *(Source: Adapted from IDSA/ESMO recommendations [1, 5])*

Type of sample	Modalities	Purpose	Notes
Blood cultures *(Systematic*	• **2 pairs** (1 aerobic + 1 anaerobic per site)	To detect bacteremia/fungemia	• Positivity: 10-30% of NF

)	• **With CVC**: 1 pair on each lumen + 1 peripheral • **Without CVC**: 2 peripheral pairs • Volume: **8-10 mL/site** (adult)		• DTP > 2h (CVC vs periphery) Infection catheter-related
ECBU ***(Systematic)***	• 2nd stream of urine or urinary catheter (not the bag) • Vulvar/urethral cleansing before sampling	To diagnose an asymptomatic urinary tract infection	• Culture if leucocyturia > 10^4/mL • Look for *C. difficile* if diarrhoea
Directed sampling			
ENT/Pulmonary area	• **Throat**: angina/pharyngitis • **ECBC** (sputum) • **BAL** if pneumonia • **Viral PCR** (nasopharyngeal): Influenza/RSV/COVID	Identify pneumopathies/viral infections	• BAL reserved for severe or undiagnosed pneumonia • Multiplex PCR recommended
Digestive tract	• **Coproculture** + *C. difficile* toxins • **PCR enteropathogens** (Norovirus, etc.)	Infectious diarrhoea	• *C. difficile* frequently treated with ATB • Strict isolation if positive
Skin/Tissue Mosquitoes	- **Swab** skin lesion - **Puncture** collection/abscess - **Biopsy** if deep lesion	Detect cellulitis/abscess/fungemia	• Add direct examination (Gram, Giemsa) • Fungal culture if suspected
CSF	• **Lumbar puncture** (after imaging if neurological signs) • Analysis: Cytology/biochemistry/viral PCR/culture	Meningitis/encephalitis	• Contraindications: HTIC/coagulation disorders • PCR herpes/EBV/CMV if immunocompromised
Other	• **Joint puncture** (arthritis) • **Ascites** (biochemical analysis/culture)	Localised infections	- Adapted to the clinical context

Optimal blood culture strategy

1. **Technique** :

○ Skin disinfection (alcohol+ povidone iodine/chlorhexidine).

○ Do not change needles after sampling.

2. **Interpretation** :

○ **DTP (Difference in Positivity Time)**:

■ CVC > Periphery of > **2h** Catheter-related infection.

○ **Contamination** :

■ *Staphylococcus epidermidis* or *Cutibacterium*: Check the clinic.

4.3 Initial imaging: Locating the source of infection

The aim of imaging is to locate a deep-seated infection, particularly in the lungs or abdomen, which may not be obvious clinically.

- **4.3.1 Chest X-ray: Systematic but of limited sensitivity**
  - A frontal chest X-ray (and profile if possible) should be performed **systematically as an emergency** in any febrile neutropenic patient, even in the absence of respiratory symptoms [1, 5].
  - It may reveal pneumopathy (alveolar condensation, interstitial infiltrate), pleural effusion or mediastinal adenopathy.
  - However, its **sensitivity is limited** in neutropenic patients, as the inflammatory response is attenuated and radiological signs of incipient pneumonitis may be absent or delayed. A normal radiograph does not therefore rule out pulmonary infection.
- **4.3.2 Other imaging tests (depending on the clinical presentation or persistence of fever):**
  - **Thoracic computed tomography (CT) :**
    - Indications: Persistent or worsening respiratory symptoms despite a normal X-ray, suspicion of a pulmonary focus not visible on X-ray, unexplained persistent fever after 48-72h of antibiotic therapy.
    - Much more sensitive than X-ray for detecting incipient pulmonary infiltrates, nodules (aspergillosis?), minimal pleural effusions and adenopathy. Helps to guide a possible BAL.
  - **Abdominopelvic CT:**
    - Indications: Abdominal pain, profuse or bloody diarrhoea, suspected colitis (neutropenic enterocolitis/typhlitis), intra-abdominal abscess, pancreatitis, or unexplained persistent fever.
  - **Abdominal ultrasound:**
    - May be useful in the first instance to clear up abdominal pain (look for cholecystitis, liver abscess, appendicitis, hydronephrosis).
  - **Brain MRI:**
    - If central neurological signs (see Chapter 3).
  - **Other (more rarely as an initial emergency):** Labelled leucocyte scintigraphy (if prolonged fever and focus not found), PET scan (especially for follow-up or to look for deep fungal foci).

Conclusion

Emergency paraclinical examinations of febrile neutropenic patients are essential for confirming the diagnosis, assessing the severity of the situation, and attempting to identify a pathogenic agent and an infectious site. A full biological work-up, systematic blood cultures combined with clinically-directed sampling, and a chest X-ray are the key elements of this initial assessment. Procalcitonin can provide diagnostic assistance, while more advanced imaging tests such as chest or abdominal CT scans are reserved for specific indications. All this data, together with clinical information, will enable the patient's risk to be stratified and the most appropriate empirical antibiotic therapy to be initiated, which will be the subject of the next chapter.

References

1. Freifeld AG, Bow EJ, Sepkowitz KA, et al. Clinical practice guideline for the use of antimicrobial agents in neutropenic patients with cancer: 2010 update by the Infectious Diseases Society of America. Clin Infect Dis. 2011;52(4):e56-e93.

2. Van der Velden WJ, Blijlevens NM, Feuth T, et al. The predictive value of C-reactive protein and procalcitonin in a cohort of 205 febrile neutropenic patients with a hematological malignancy. Support Care Cancer. 2010;18(1):65-71.

3. Póvoa P, Salluh JI, Martinez ML, Guillamat-Prats R, Soares M, Nseir S, Koulenti D, Rello J; ESEPTIC Co-operative Study Group. Clinical impact of procalcitonin in patients with sepsis: a prospective, multicenter, randomized, controlled trial. Crit Care. 2011 Dec 8;15(6):R270.

4. Schuetz P, Beishuizen A, Broyles M, et al. Procalcitonin (PCT)-guided antibiotic stewardship: an international multidisciplinary consensus on optimized clinical use. Clin Chem Lab Med. 2017;55(10):1427-1439.

5. Klastersky J, de Naurois J, Rolston K, et al. Management of febrile neutropaenia: ESMO Clinical Practice Guidelines. Ann Oncol. 2016;27(suppl 5):v111-v118.

6. Mermel LA, Allon M, Bouza E, et al. Clinical practice guidelines for the diagnosis and management of intravascular catheter-related infection: 2009 Update by the Infectious Diseases Society of America. Clin Infect Dis. 2009;49(1):1-45.

Chapter 5: Risk Stratification and Prognostic Scoring in Febrile Neutropenia

Introduction

Not all episodes of febrile neutropenia (NF) carry the same risk of serious complications or mortality. A crucial step after the initial diagnosis is therefore to **stratify** the patient's **risk.** The aim is to identify "low-risk" patients who could benefit from simplified management (sometimes outpatient with oral antibiotic therapy), and "high-risk" patients requiring hospitalisation and aggressive intravenous antibiotic therapy [1]. Several prognostic scores have been developed and validated to help with this stratification. This chapter details the principles of risk assessment, presents the MASCC score (the most widely used), discusses other relevant scores, and discusses the implications of this stratification on initial treatment decisions.

5.1 Principles of Risk Stratification: Why and How?

- **5.1.1 Objectives of Risk Stratification :**

  - **Optimise the use of resources:** Avoid unnecessary hospitalisations and broad-spectrum intravenous antibiotic therapy for low-risk patients, thereby reducing costs, exposure to nosocomial infections and antibiotic selection pressure.
  - **Intensify monitoring and treatment for high-risk patients:** Ensure rapid and aggressive management for those most likely to develop serious complications.
  - **Personalise management:** adapt the therapeutic strategy (place of care, type of antibiotics) to the patient's individual risk profile.

- **5.1.2 General criteria for identifying high-risk patients:** Independently of the scores, certain clinical and paraclinical criteria identified during the initial assessment (see Chapters 3 and 4) immediately classify a patient as being at high risk of complications [2, 3]. These include (but are not limited to)

  - Profound (PNN < 0.1 G/L) and/or prolonged neutropenia expected (> 7 days).
  - Signs of severe sepsis or septic shock (hypotension, tachycardia, altered consciousness, etc.).
  - Significant uncontrolled co-morbidities (severe renal/hepatic failure, decompensated heart failure, symptomatic COPD).
  - Severe clinically evident infection (pneumonitis, extensive cellulitis, complicated catheter infection).
  - Grade 3-4 mucositis.

o Rapid progression of symptoms.
o Patient hospitalised at time of onset of fever.
o Recent haematopoietic stem cell allograft. These patients require hospitalisation and aggressive management, and the calculation of a prognostic score has less impact on the initial decision to hospitalise.

5.2 The MASCC Score (Multinational Association for Supportive Care in Cancer)

The MASCC score is the most widely used and validated risk stratification tool for identifying febrile neutropenic patients at low risk of serious medical complications [4, 5].

. 5.2.1 Calculation of the MASCC Score :

The score is calculated from seven clinical and paraclinical variables assessed at the patient's initial presentation (see Table 5.1). A total score is obtained by adding the points allocated to each variable.
The maximum score is 26 points.

Tableau 1 1: Calculation of the MASCC score

(Source: Adapted from references [4, 5])

Variable	Criteria	Points awarded
1. Severity of symptoms	Absence or mild symptoms	**5**
	Moderate symptoms	**3**
	Severe symptoms (e.g. confusion, distress) respiratory distress)	**0**
2. Systolic blood pressure	SAP > 90 mmHg	**5**
	SBP < 90 mmHg	**0**
3. No COPD	No history of COPD	**4**
	Known COPD	**0**
4. Type of cancer	Solid tumour **or** haemopathy without previous invasive fungal infection	**4**
	Haemopathy with previous fungal infection	**0**
5. Hydration	No dehydration requiring IV fluids	**3**
	Dehydration requiring IV rehydration	**0**
6. Ambulatory status	Patient ambulatory at onset of fever	**4**
	Non-ambulatory patient (bedridden/hospitalised)	**0**
7. Age	< 60 years old	**2**
	> *60* years old	**0**

- 5.2.2 Interpretation of the MASCC score :

- **MASCC Score > 21:** Defines a patient at **low risk of** serious complications (risk < 5-10%). These patients may be eligible for outpatient management or short hospitalisation with short-term oral or IV antibiotic therapy, under certain conditions (see section 5.4).
- **MASCC Score < 21:** Defines a patient at **high risk of** serious complications. These patients require hospitalisation and intravenous antibiotic therapy.

Tableau 2 2: Interpretation and clinical application of the MASCC score

(Source: Adapted from Klastersky et al [4] and ASCO/IDSA recommendations [2, 3])

Score MASCC	Level of Risk	Risk of Complications	Management Recommended	Monitoring
> 21	Low risk	< 5-10%	**Option 1**: Management outpatient with oral ATB (e.g. daily + : Ciprofloxacin +) D2-J4 Amoxicillin/clavulanic acid) **Option 2**: Short hospital stay (24-48 hours) then oral relay if improvement	Consultation CBC at
< 21	High risk	> 20%	Immediate hospitalisation + Broad-spectrum IV ATB (eg: Piperacillin-Tazobactam or Cefepime)	Monitoring continuous (scope, diuresis) + markers inflammatory markers

Figure 5.1: Algorithm for using the MASCC score

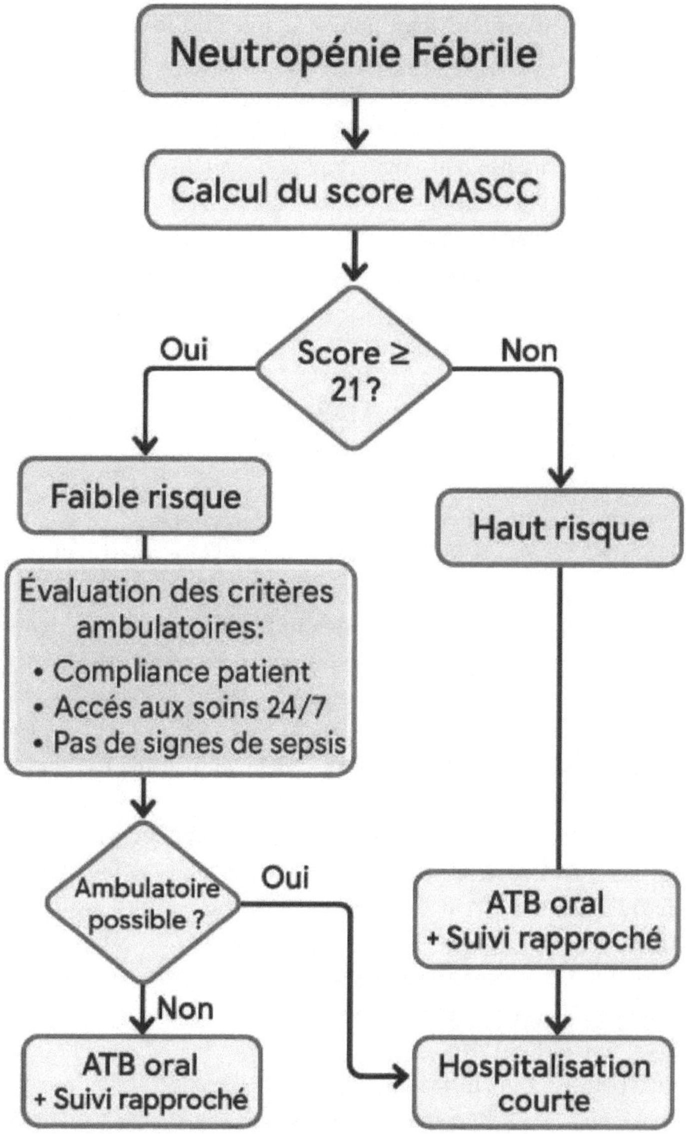

- 5.2.3 Usefulness and limitations of the MASCC score :

○ **Usefulness :**

■ Simple tool, quick to calculate, and well validated in numerous studies.

■ Helps to objectively identify patients who could benefit from less intensive management.

■ Standardises practices and facilitates clinical research.

○ **Limitations:**

■ The 21-point threshold may not be applicable to all populations or all contexts (e.g. certain haematological malignancies).

■ Clinical judgement remains essential: a patient with a score > *21* but presenting certain signs of severity not taken into account by the score (e.g. severe mucositis, intense pain) may require hospitalisation.

■ Does not take into account the expected duration of neutropenia, which is an important prognostic factor.

■ Requires a full initial assessment and the availability of certain biological results.

■ Its performance may be poorer in certain specific situations (e.g. fungal or viral infections).

It is therefore crucial to use the MASCC score as a decision-making tool, always integrating it with an overall clinical assessment and the physician's judgement [5, 6].

5.3 Other Prognostic Scores and Clinical Approaches

Although the MASCC score is the most widely used, other tools and approaches exist.

- **5.3.1 CISNE Score (Clinical Index of Stable Febrile Neutropenia):**

Developed more recently, the CISNE score also aims to identify low-risk patients by focusing on easily accessible clinical variables, particularly in patients with solid tumours [7]. It incorporates factors such as ECOG status, cardiovascular stress, chronic COPD, grade >2 mucositis, and monocytic neutropenia.

○ It stratifies patients into three risk categories (low, intermediate, high).

○ It is less widely used than the MASCC but offers an alternative, particularly when the MASCC seems less discriminating.

- **5.3.2 Scores Specific to Certain Populations:**

Scores adapted to specific populations (e.g. acute leukaemia patients, transplant recipients) may exist or be under development.

- **5.3.3 Clinical Gestalt:**

Even in the absence of formal scores, the experience and clinical judgement of the physician, based on the overall assessment of the patient (severity of symptoms, comorbidities, speed of progression, social and environmental support), play a fundamental role in risk stratification [1, 3]. Many experienced clinicians can intuitively identify high-risk patients. However, scores provide useful objectivity and standardisation.

Table 5.3: Comparison of MASCC and CISNE scores
(Source: Adapted from references [1, 3, 7])

Characteristic	MASCC score	CISNE score
Target population	All cancers (solid + haemopathies)	Mainly solid tumours
Variables included	• General symptoms • NOT • COPD • Type of cancer • Hydration • Ambulatory status -Age	• ECOG status • Cardiovascular stress • COPD • Mucositis > Grade 2 • Monocytic neutropenia
Risk thresholds	- Low risk: > 21 - High risk: < 21	- Low risk: 0 points - Intermediate: 1-2 points - High risk: > 3 points
Benefits	- Broad validation - Simple to calculate	• Better discrimination for solid tumours • Incorporates ECOG and mucositis
Limitations	Less accurate for tumours diseases	Not validated for solid
Recommended use	Standard for all patients	Alternative for solid tumours at ambiguous risk with MASCC

5.4 Implication of Risk Stratification on Initial Therapeutic Decisions

Risk stratification has direct implications for initial therapeutic choices, including the place of care and the type of empirical antibiotic therapy [1, 2, 3, 6].

- 5.4.1 Low-risk patients (e.g. MASCC score > 21 AND no clinical severity criteria) :

○ **Outpatient management possible UNDER STRICT CONDITIONS :**

■ Absence of severe uncontrolled comorbidities.

■ Satisfactory renal and hepatic function.

■ Good general condition, patient able to take oral medication.

■ Easy access to a care centre in case of worsening (geographical proximity, telephone).

■ Good family and environmental support.

■ Possibility of close clinical and biological monitoring (consultation or telephone call on D1-D2, follow-up CBC).

■ Patient and family educated and cooperative.

○ **Empirical oral antibiotic therapy:** Combination of a fluoroquinolone (e.g. ciprofloxacin or levofloxacin) AND amoxicillin-clavulanic acid (or clindamycin if allergic to penicillins) [3].

○ If a short initial hospital stay is preferred: initial IV antibiotic therapy (e.g. ceftriaxone), followed by an early oral relay if improvement is seen.

- **5.4.2 High-risk patients (e.g. MASCC score < 21 OR presence of clinical severity criteria) :**

  - **Systematic hospitalisation.**
  - **Empirical broad-spectrum intravenous antibiotic therapy** (see Chapter 6 for specific choices).
  - Intensive monitoring and frequent reassessment.

- **5.4.3 Intermediate or Doubtful cases :**

In the event of a borderline score, discordance between score and clinical impression, or if certain conditions for outpatient treatment are not met, it is more prudent to opt for initial hospitalisation and close monitoring. Reassessment at H24-H48 may allow early discharge to be reconsidered if the outcome is favourable.

Table 5.4: Therapeutic implications according to risk stratification in febrile neutropenia

(Source: Adapted from IDSA/ASCO/ESMO guidelines [1-3, 6])

Stratification	**Place of care**	**Initial antibiotic therapy**	**Monitoring**
Low risk (MASCC >21 + no severity criteria)	**Ambulatory** (if strict conditions are met)	**Oral** : • Ciprofloxacin (500 mg x2/d)+ Amoxicillin/Ac clav (1g x3/d) • Alternative: Levofloxacin (750 mg/d) if allergic to ß-lactams	- Consultation/J1-J2 • CBC at 48 hours • Alert for persistent fever >48h
High risk (MASCC <21 or severity criteria)	**Systematic hospitalisation**	**Broad-spectrum IV** : - Piperacillin-Tazobactam (4.5g x3/d) • Cefepime (2g x3/d) • Carbapenem (if risk of Pseudomonas/Resistance)	• Continuous monitoring (scope, diuresis) • CRP/PCT at 2448h • Daily clinical reassessment
Intermediate cases (MASCC borderline or clinical doubt)	**Initial hospitalisation**	**Initial IV** (eg: Ceftriaxone 2g/d) then oral relay if improvement at 48h	- Reassessment at H24-H48 to adapt strategy

Risk stratification is a dynamic process that must be reassessed according to the patient's clinical progress.

Conclusion

Risk stratification is a fundamental and early stage in the management of febrile neutropenia. It makes it possible to adapt the intensity of care to the profile of each patient, identifying those who can be treated safely on an outpatient basis and those who require hospitalisation and aggressive antibiotic therapy. The MASCC score is the most validated tool for this approach, but it must always be interpreted in the light of clinical judgement and patient specificities. Accurate risk stratification helps not only to improve the prognosis of high-risk patients, but also to optimise healthcare resources and preserve the quality of life of low-risk patients. Initial therapeutic decisions, particularly the choice of empirical antibiotic therapy, will be a direct result of this risk assessment, as will be detailed in the next chapter.

References

1. Klastersky J, de Naurois J, Rolston K, et al. Management of febrile neutropaenia: ESMO Clinical Practice Guidelines. Ann Oncol. 2016;27(suppl 5):v111-v118.

2. Taplitz RA, Kennedy EB, Bow EJ, et al. Outpatient Management of Febrile Neutropenia in Adults Treated for Malignancy: American Society of Clinical Oncology and Infectious Diseases Society of America Clinical Practice Guideline Update. J Clin Oncol. 2018;36(14):1443-1453.

3. Freifeld AG, Bow EJ, Sepkowitz KA, et al. Clinical practice guideline for the use of antimicrobial agents in neutropenic patients with cancer: 2010 update by the Infectious Diseases Society of America. Clin Infect Dis. 2011;52(4):e56-e93.

4. Klastersky J, Paesmans M, Rubenstein EB, et al. The Multinational Association for Supportive Care in Cancer risk index: A multinational scoring system for identifying low-risk febrile neutropenic cancer patients. J Clin Oncol. 2000;18(16):3038-3051.

5. Uys A, Rapoport BL, Anderson R. Febrile neutropenia: aetiology, risk factors and treatment. S Afr Med J. 2004;94(8 Pt 2):681-687.

6. Ahn S, Lee YS, Chun YH, et al. The MASCC risk index for febrile neutropenia: a meta-analysis. Support Care Cancer. 2013;21(5):1487-1492.

7. Carmona-Bayonas A, Jiménez-Fonseca P, Virizuela Echaburu J, et al. Prediction of serious complications in patients with seemingly stable febrile neutropenia: validation of the Clinical Index of Stable Febrile Neutropenia (CISNE) in a prospective cohort. J Clin Oncol. 2015;33(5):480-486.

Part 3

Therapeutic Management

Chapter 6: Principles of Initial Empirical Antibiotic Therapy in Febrile Neutropenia

Introduction

Once the diagnosis of febrile neutropenia (NF) has been made and the patient's risk stratified, the rapid initiation of appropriate empirical antibiotic therapy is the cornerstone of management and a major determinant of prognosis [1]. In the absence of an obvious infection or initial microbiological documentation, this antibiotic therapy aims to cover the most likely and most virulent pathogens. The choice of drug should be guided by clinical severity, risk stratification, local epidemiology of bacterial resistance, and the patient's specific characteristics. This chapter describes the urgency of initiation, the objectives of empirical antibiotic therapy, strategies for choosing antibiotics for low- and high-risk patients, and the role of glycopeptides as first-line antibiotics.

6.1 The Golden Hour of Initiation

The concept of "The Golden Hour", well known in the management of sepsis and septic shock, is fully applicable to febrile neutropenia, particularly in high-risk patients [2, 3].

- **Risk of rapid progression to sepsis:** In neutropenic patients, a bacterial infection may progress very rapidly to severe sepsis or septic shock due to the absence of effective neutrophil defences.
- **Impact of delay in administration on mortality:** Numerous studies have shown that a delay in administration of the first dose of antibiotics after recognition of NF (or sepsis) is associated with a significant increase in mortality [2, 4]. Every hour of delay can count.
- **Objective: Administration within one hour of recognition of NF and completion of microbiological sampling (if possible).**
  - This requires optimum organisation of emergency departments, oncology/haematology units and hospital pharmacies, with clear protocols and rapidly available antibiotics.
  - Microbiological samples (particularly blood cultures) should be taken before the first dose of antibiotics, but should never delay the start of treatment.

should **never delay** the initiation of treatment if the patient presents signs of severity.

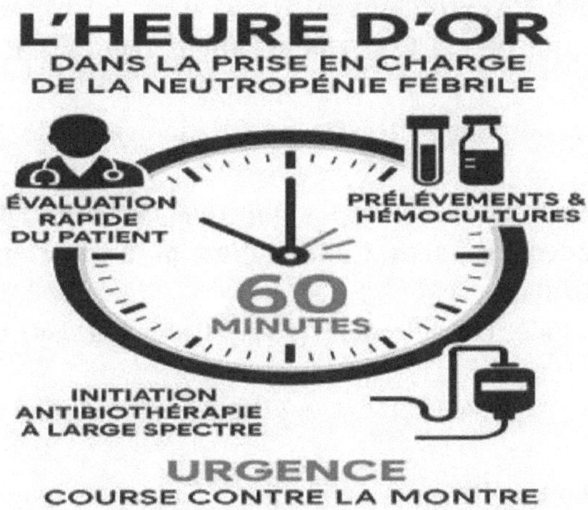
L'HEURE D'OR
DANS LA PRISE EN CHARGE
DE LA NEUTROPÉNIE FÉBRILE
ÉVALUATION
RAPIDE
DU PATIENT
PRÉLÈVEMENTS &
HÉMOCULTURES
60
MINUTES
INITIATION
ANTIBIOTHÉRAPIE
À LARGE SPECTRE
URGENCE
COURSE CONTRE LA MONTRE

Figure 6.1: Schematic representation of "The Golden Hour" in the management of febrile neutropenia, highlighting the urgency of assessment, sampling and initiation of antibiotic therapy.

6.2 Objectives of Empirical Antibiotic Therapy

Initial empirical antibiotic therapy aims to [1, 3, 5] :

- **Cover the bacterial pathogens most frequently responsible for severe and rapidly progressive infections** in neutropenic patients, in particular Gram-negative bacilli (GNB) such as *Pseudomonas aeruginosa* and Enterobacteriaceae, as well as certain virulent Gram-positive cocci (GPC).
- **Rapidly obtain effective antibiotic concentrations** at the site of infection (presumed or proven).
- **Reduce the morbidity and mortality** associated with bacterial infection.
- **Prevent the development of complications** such as septic shock or organ failure.
- Allow the patient to **stabilise clinically** while awaiting the results of microbiological cultures, which can guide any adaptation or de-escalation of treatment.

It is important to note that initial empirical antibiotic therapy does not generally target fungal or viral infections, except in very specific clinical situations (see Chapters 8 and 9).

6.3 Choice of molecules according to risk stratification and local epidemiology

The choice of empirical antibiotic therapy is guided by the patient's risk stratification (low risk vs high risk, see Chapter 5) and must take account of local epidemiological data concerning prevalent pathogens and their antibiotic susceptibility profiles [1, 3, 5].

- 6.3.1 Patients at low risk of complications (e.g. MASCC score > 21, clinically stable)

○ **Criteria for outpatient treatment (if all conditions are met - see Chapter 5.4.1):**

■ These patients may be eligible for **empirical oral antibiotic therapy**.

■ **Recommended regimen: Combination of a fluoroquinolone AND amoxicillin-clavulanic acid** [3, 5].

■ Fluoroquinolone: Ciprofloxacin (500-750 mg x 2/day) or Levofloxacin (500-750 mg x 1/day).

■ Amoxicillin-clavulanic acid: 875mg/125mg x 2-3/day or 500mg/125mg x 3/day.

■ In cases of true allergy to penicillins: Fluoroquinolone + Clindamycin (300-450mg x 3- 4/day).

■ The first dose can sometimes be administered IV in hospital before discharge.

■ Close clinical and biological monitoring is essential (consultation or telephone contact on D1-D2, follow-up blood count).

○ **If hospital treatment for a low-risk patient:**

■ Initial IV antibiotic therapy (e.g. ceftriaxone, piperacillin- tazobactam at an appropriate dose) with the possibility of early oral relay (after 24-48h if apyrexia and clinical stability).

- 6.3.2 Patients at high risk of complications (e.g. MASCC score < 21 or signs of severity)

○ **Systematic hospitalisation.**

○ **Intravenous broad-spectrum bactericidal antibiotics with anti-pseudomonas activity.**

○ Several options are available, the choice depending on the local epidemiology, the patient's history (BMR colonisation/infection), the clinical severity and any allergies.

○ **Monotherapy :**

■ **Piperacillin-tazobactam (4g/0.5g IV every 6-8 hours)**: Often the first-line choice in many centres. Broad spectrum including *P. aeruginosa*, most enterobacteria, and activity on some anaerobes and CGPs.

■ **Cefepime (2g IV every 8 hours)**: Broad-spectrum 4th generation cephalosporin , good antipseudomonas activity.

■ **Ceftazidime (2g IV every 8 hours)**: 3rd generation anti-pseudomonas cephalosporin. Less commonly used as monotherapy due to reduced coverage of CGP and risk of emergence of ESBL.

■ **Carbapenems (Imipenem-cilastatin 500mg IV every 6 hours, Meropenem 1g IV every 8 hours)**: Very broad-spectrum antibiotics, including *P. aeruginosa* and most extended-spectrum beta-lactamase (ESBL)-producing enterobacteria. Their first-line use should be **reserved** for specific situations to limit the emergence of resistance (carbapenemases):

■ Patients with severe sepsis or septic shock.

■ Colonisation or previous documented infection with ESBL-producing bacteria.

■ Local epidemiology with high prevalence of ESBL.

■ Failure of first-line antibiotic therapy.

○ **Dual therapy:**

■ **Combination of an anti-pseudomonas beta-lactam (piperacillin-tazobactam, cefepime, ceftazidime, carbapenem) AND an aminoglycoside (amikacin, gentamicin, tobramycin) OR an anti-pseudomonas fluoroquinolone (ciprofloxacin, levofloxacin IV).**

■ **Potential advantages:** Bactericidal synergy, broader spectrum, prevention of the emergence of resistance (especially with aminoglycosides).

■ **Disadvantages:** Risk of increased toxicity (nephrotoxicity and ototoxicity of aminoglycosides), little demonstration of clinical superiority over appropriate monotherapy in most situations [1, 5, 6].

■ **Indications for dual therapy (often with an aminoglycoside for the first 48-72 hours):**

■ Patients with severe sepsis or septic shock.

■ Strong suspicion or documentation of infection with *P. aeruginosa* or other difficult BGN.

■ Local epidemiology with high rates of resistance to beta-lactams alone.

■ Patient with high mortality risk factors.

Table 6.1: Options for empirical antibiotic therapy in febrile neutropenia

(Source: Adapted from IDSA/ESMO/ASCO guidelines [1, 3, 5])

Stratification	Recommended Regimen	Spectrum of Activity	Standard Dosage	Remarks
Low risk (ambulatory)	Ciprofloxacin + Amoxicillin/Ac clavulanic prophylaxis	BGN (except Pseudomonas), CGP	- Cipro: 500-750 mg x2/d PO - Amox/Clav: 875/125 mg x2/d PO	Contraindicated if prophylaxis by fluoroquinolone
High risk (monotherapy IV MONOTHERAPY)	Piperacillin-Tazobactam	BGN (including Pseudomonas), CGP, anaerobes	4.5 g x3-4/d IV	1st line choice in most centres
	Cefepime	BGN (including Pseudomonas), CGP	2 g x3/d IV	Alternative to Pip-Taz
	Meropenem	BGN (including ESBL), Pseudomonas,	1 g x3/d IV	Reserved for risks of ESBL/septic

		anaerobes		shock
High risk (dual IV therapy)	Pip-Taz+ Amikacin	Broader spectrum (antiPseudomonas synergy)	- Pip-Taz : 4.5 g x3/d IV - Amikacin: 15-20 mg/kg/d IV	48-72h then re-evaluation
	Cefepime+ Cipro floxacin	Enhanced Pseudomonas coverage	• Cefepime: 2 g x3/d IV • Cipro: 400 mg x2/d	If allergic to aminoglycosides

Figure 6.2: Decision tree for high-risk empirical antibiotic therapy

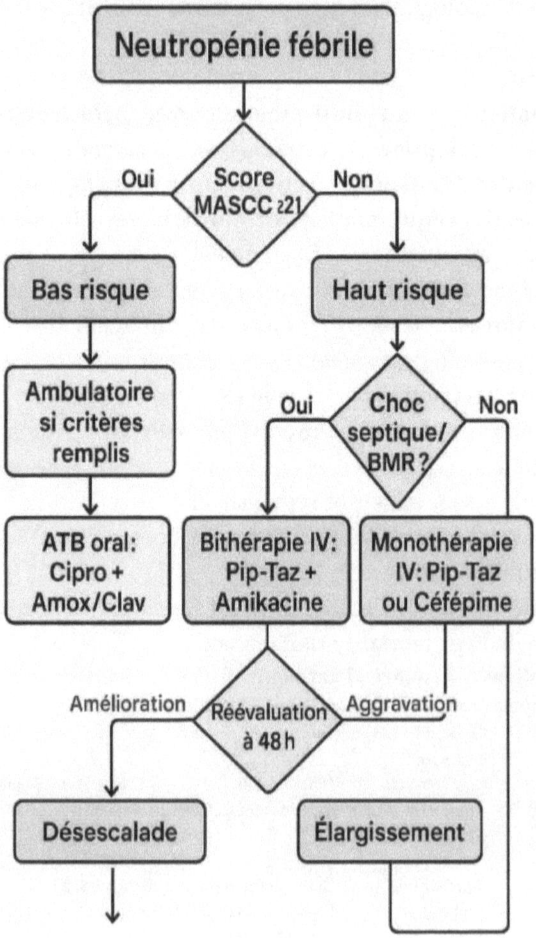

- **BMR**: Multi-resistant bacteria

6.4 Place of glycopeptides (Vancomycin, Teicoplanin) as First-line treatment

The systematic addition of a glycopeptide (e.g. vancomycin) to initial empirical antibiotic therapy to cover resistant Gram-positive cocci (particularly MRSA - methicillin-resistant *Staphylococcus aureus*) **is NOT recommended in the absence of a specific indication** [1, 3, 5].

- **Reasons :**

o Increased costs.

o Risk of side-effects (nephrotoxicity, "Red Man Syndrome" with vancomycin).

o Selection pressure favouring the emergence of vancomycin-resistant enterococci (VRE).

o Little impact on overall mortality when used systematically.

- **Restrictive indications for adding a glycopeptide as a first-line treatment:**

o **Strong clinical suspicion of infection related to the central venous catheter** (inflammatory signs at the insertion site, chills during infusion on the catheter).

o **Severe skin or soft tissue infection** (extensive cellulitis, abscess).

o **Previous documented MRSA or VRE colonisation** (if VRE is susceptible to vancomycin/teicoplanin, otherwise other agents such as linezolid or daptomycin would be discussed).

o **Severe sepsis or septic shock** (pending microbiological results, for maximum coverage).

o **Radiologically documented pneumonia** (some protocols include this, but it is debatable).

o Persistent hypotension despite well-administered anti-BGN antibiotics.

- If a glycopeptide is initiated empirically, it should be **reassessed at 48-72 hours** according to the microbiological results and the clinical course, and discontinued if there is no documentation of infection with CGP to justify it.

6.5 Adaptation of Dosages to Renal and Hepatic Function

Many antibiotics are eliminated by the kidneys. It is therefore crucial to adapt their dosage to the patient's creatinine clearance to avoid toxic accumulation or, conversely, under-dosing.

- **Assessment of renal function:** Calculation of creatinine clearance (Cockcroft-Gault formula or MDRD/CKD-EPI) before initiation and during treatment.
- **Antibiotics requiring dose adjustment in cases of renal impairment:**

o Beta-lactams (penicillins, cephalosporins, carbapenems): most require dose

reduction or interval spacing.
◦ Aminosides: strict adjustment according to residual levels and renal function (major risk of nephrotoxicity and ototoxicity).
◦ Glycopeptides (vancomycin, teicoplanin): adjustment according to residual levels and renal function.
◦ Fluoroquinolones (some).
- **Antibiotics with mainly hepatic elimination:**
◦ Certain macrolides, clindamycin, metronidazole, rifampicin. Adaptation may be necessary in cases of severe hepatic impairment.
- It is essential to refer to the specific recommendations (drug SPC, pharmacological databases) for the dosage adjustment of each antibiotic.

Conclusion

Initiation of empirical antibiotic therapy is a critical and urgent step in the management of febrile neutropenia. Adherence to the "golden hour" concept is fundamental to improving the prognosis of patients, particularly those at high risk. The choice of antibiotic molecules should be guided by a rigorous risk stratification, the local epidemiology of resistance, clinical severity and patient characteristics, while aiming for broad coverage of the most likely pathogens. The use of glycopeptides as a first-line treatment must remain restrictive and justified. Lastly, adapting doses to renal function is an essential safety measure. Early re-evaluation of this empirical antibiotic therapy in the light of clinical and microbiological data, which will be discussed in the next chapter, is just as crucial for optimising treatment and limiting selection pressure.

References

1. Freifeld AG, Bow EJ, Sepkowitz KA, et al. Clinical practice guideline for the use of antimicrobial agents in neutropenic patients with cancer: 2010 update by the Infectious Diseases Society of America. Clin Infect Dis. 2011;52(4):e56-e93.
2. Rhodes A, Evans LE, Alhazzani W, et al. Surviving Sepsis Campaign: International Guidelines for Management of Sepsis and Septic Shock: 2016. Crit Care Med. 2017;45(3):486-552.
3. Taplitz RA, Kennedy EB, Bow EJ, et al. Outpatient Management of Febrile Neutropenia in Adults Treated for Malignancy: American Society of Clinical Oncology and Infectious Diseases Society of America Clinical Practice Guideline Update. J Clin Oncol. 2018;36(14):1443-1453.
4. Kumar A, Roberts D, Wood KE, et al. Duration of hypotension before initiation of effective antimicrobial therapy is the critical determinant of survival in human septic shock. Crit Care Med. 2006;34(6):1589-1596.

5. Klastersky J, de Naurois J, Rolston K, et al. Management of febrile neutropaenia: ESMO Clinical Practice Guidelines. Ann Oncol. 2016;27(suppl 5):v111-v118.
6. Paul M, Dickstein Y, Borok S, Leibovici L, Yahav D. Beta-lactam monotherapy versus beta-lactam-aminoglycoside combination therapy for sepsis in immunocompetent patients: a meta-analysis of randomized trials. Antimicrob Agents Chemother. 2014 Mar;58(3):1768.

Chapter 7: Reassessment and Adaptation of Antibiotic Therapy in Febrile Neutropenia

Introduction

The prompt initiation of empirical broad-spectrum antibiotic therapy is a vital measure in the initial management of febrile neutropenia (NF). However, this strategy must be followed by a rigorous clinical and biological reassessment, typically between 48 and 72 hours (H48-H72), or even sooner in the event of worsening. The purpose of this reassessment is to assess the effectiveness of the initial treatment, to identify any infectious sites or specific pathogens on the basis of the results of the initial samples, and to adapt the antibiotic strategy accordingly. The aim is to optimise efficacy while limiting selection pressure, side effects and costs, in particular by de-escalation strategies where possible [1, 2]. This chapter details the reassessment process, explores the different clinical scenarios and the resulting therapeutic adaptations, and discusses the principles guiding the duration of antibiotic treatment.

7.1 Systematic reassessment at H48-H72: a key moment

The period from 48 to 72 hours after initiation of empirical antibiotic therapy is a critical milestone in the management of NF [3, 4].

- **Objectives of the reassessment :**

    - Assess the clinical response to the initial antibiotic treatment (changes in fever, vital signs, local symptoms).
    - Analyse the results of the initial microbiological samples (blood cultures, ECBU, other directed samples).
    - Look for an infectious outbreak that may not have been identified initially.
    - Reassess the patient's risk stratification.
    - Decide whether to continue, modify or stop certain antibiotics (de-escalation).
    - Consider the need for further investigations (imaging, new samples).

- **Elements of the reassessment :**

    - **Clinical:** Temperature, general condition, vital signs, full clinical examination to look for the appearance of or changes in signs of infection.
    - **Biological:** New CBC (change in PNN), CRP (expected to fall if there has been a favourable response to bacterial infection), renal and liver function (tolerance of antibiotics). Procalcitonin if initially measured (its kinetics may be informative) [5].
    - **Microbiology**: results of blood cultures (positivity, germ identification, antibiogram), ECBU and other cultures.
    - **Imaging:** reinterpretation of the initial chest X-ray, CT scan if indicated (e.g. unexplained persistent fever, new pulmonary signs).

7.2 Management of different clinical and biological scenarios at H48-H72

Therapeutic adaptation will depend on the clinical course and microbiological results.

- **7.2.1 Scenario 1: Apyretic and Clinically Stable Patient, Unidentified Outbreak, Negative Cultures**

  - This is the most common situation in low-risk patients who have responded well.
  - **Management:**
    - If initially low-risk patient treated orally as an outpatient: continue the same treatment for a total of 5-7 days or until resolution of neutropenia (PNN >0.5 G/L for >48h), according to Involution [3].
    - In initially high-risk patients admitted to hospital:
    - Possibility **of therapeutic de-escalation** (see section 7.3).
    - Switch to oral antibiotic therapy (oral relay) if the criteria are met (clinical stability, digestive tolerance, PNN in recovery phase, no deep focus requiring prolonged IV treatment).
    - IV antibiotic therapy continued until resolution of neutropenia and apyrexia for >48 hours.

- **7.2.2 Scenario 2: Apyretic and Clinically Stable Patient, Identified Outbreak and/or Positive Microbiological Documentation**

  - **Management :**
    - **Adaptation of antibiotic therapy to the antibiogram of** the germ identified (if available). This is the **targeted de-escalation** stage: choosing the narrowest and most appropriate antibiotic.
    - If the germ is sensitive to the initial empirical antibiotic therapy, this can be continued or simplified (e.g. switching from dual therapy to monotherapy).
    - The duration of treatment should be adapted to the site of infection and the pathogen (e.g. 7-14 days for BGN bacteremia, longer for osteoarticular infection or endocarditis).
    - If catheter-related infection: discuss removal of the catheter and adapt antibiotic therapy (see Chapter 15).

- **7.2.3 Scenario 3: Persistent Febrile (>38°C) but Clinically Stable Patient, Unidentified Site, Negative Cultures**

  - This is a frequent situation and often a cause for concern.
  - **Complementary diagnostic approach:**
    - Thorough clinical re-examination to look for an unrecognised outbreak.
    - Repeat blood cultures (especially if shivering).
    - Thoracic CT scan (systematic if not done initially) and/or abdomino-

pelvic CT scan if there is a presenting complaint or fever >5-7 days.

■ Search for non-bacterial causes of fever: viral (PCR), fungal (galactomannan antigen, Beta-D-glucan, CT scan if prolonged neutropenia), medicinal, inflammatory (irAE, tumour progression).

○ **Therapeutic adjustment:**

■ **If no change in initial empiric antibiotic therapy (if appropriate and broad spectrum) for the first 3-5 days** if the patient remains stable, as defervescence may be delayed in the neutropenic patient.

■ **After 4-7 days of unexplained persistent fever and profound neutropenia:**

■ Add **of** an **antifungal treatment**
targeting Aspergillus and Candida (see Chapter 8) [1, 3].

■ Discuss broadening the antibacterial spectrum if not already maximal (e.g. adding coverage for anaerobes if clinically suspected, or modifying if emergence of resistance is suspected).

■ Do not systematically add a glycopeptide if there is no specific indication (see below).

- 7.2.4 Scenario 4: Persistent Febrile and/or Clinically Unstable Patient, Identified Outbreak or Positive Microbiological Documentation

○ **Management :**

■ Check that current antibiotic therapy is appropriate for the germ identified (if antibiogram available) and the location of the infection.

■ If the germ is resistant to empirical antibiotic therapy: **immediate change** to active treatment.

■ If the germ is sensitive but the patient is not improving: look for a local complication (undrained abscess, collection), spread of the infection, obstruction, or another concomitant infection. Discuss intensification of treatment (e.g. dual therapy, dose increase if possible).

■ Ensure optimal management of the outbreak (surgical drainage if abscess, removal of infected catheter, etc.).

- 7.2.5 Scenario 5: Clinical worsening (Severe Sepsis, Septic Shock) under Empirical Antibiotic Therapy

○ **Absolute therapeutic emergency.**

○ **Management in intensive care unit.**

○ **Immediate reassessment and maximum broadening of the antibiotic spectrum:**

■ Often switch to a carbapenem (if not already used) OR combination of an anti-pseudomonas beta-lactam + aminoglycoside + glycopeptide (or other anti-SARM/ERV if indicated).

- Consider anti-anaerobic coverage if abdominal or pelvic focus.
- Discuss early antifungal treatment if there are high risk factors for IFI.

o Intensive search for an uncontrolled outbreak or complication.

o Haemodynamic and respiratory support.

Figure 7.2: Algorithm for management of persistent fever or clinical worsening in the febrile neutropenic patient (Source: Adapted from IDSA/ESMO/ASCO guidelines [1, 3, 4]).

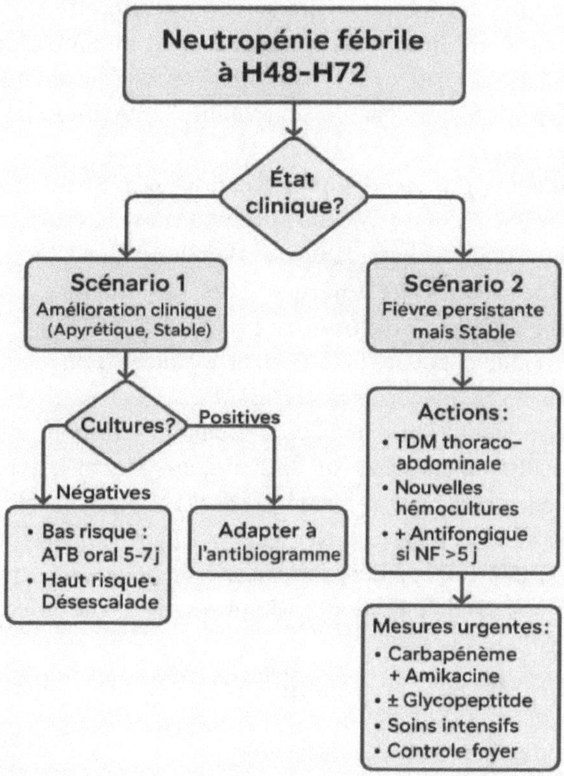

7.3 Therapeutic de-escalation strategies

Therapeutic de-escalation consists of reducing the spectrum of antibiotic therapy once clinical or microbiological information allows it. It is a key strategy in antibiotic governance to limit the emergence of resistance [1, 6].

- **Principles :**

o Possible when the patient is clinically stable or improving, and the pathogen has been identified with its susceptibility profile, or if a serious bacterial infection has been reasonably ruled out.

o Change from dual therapy to monotherapy.

o Switch from a very broad-spectrum antibiotic (e.g. carbapenem) to a narrower-spectrum antibiotic that is active against the identified germ.

o Discontinue an empirically initiated glycopeptide if there is no documentation of a CGP infection to justify it.

o Switch from an intravenous route to an oral route (oral relay) when the criteria are met (clinical stability, digestive tolerance, oral bioavailability of the antibiotic, PNN >0.5 G/L).

- **Advantages:** Reduced selection pressure, fewer side effects, lower costs.

7.4 Modification of antibiotic therapy in the event of non-response

If the patient does not respond to the initial empirical antibiotic therapy (persistent fever >3-5 days, clinical instability), modifications should be considered after a full reassessment [1, 3, 4].

- **7.4.1 Broadening the spectrum for Gram-negative bacteria :**

o If cefepime or piperacillin-tazobactam monotherapy has been used: add an aminoglycoside or an antipseudomonas fluoroquinolone, or switch to a carbapenem (especially if there is a risk of ESBL or difficult germs).

- **7.4.2 Adding an Anaerobic Blanket :**

o If an intra-abdominal, pelvic, ENT (sinusitis, Vincent's angina), necrotising skin infection or severe mucositis is suspected.

o Addition of metronidazole, or use of a beta-lactam with anti-anaerobic activity (piperacillin-tazobactam, carbapenems, amoxicillin-clavulanic acid).

- **7.4.3 Increased coverage of Gram-positive resistant cocci:**

o Addition of vancomycin (or teicoplanin) if not initiated and if signs suggestive of MRSA infection appear (catheter infection, severe pneumonia, skin infection) or if colonisation is known, or if the patient becomes haemodynamically unstable.

o If vancomycin-resistant VRE or MRSA is suspected (rare): linezolid or daptomycin.

- **7.4.4 Consider non-bacterial infection:**

o If fever persists despite appropriate broad-spectrum antibiotic therapy, and if the patient has risk factors (profound and prolonged neutropenia): **consider an invasive fungal infection** (see Chapter 8) and discuss the introduction of empirical antifungal treatment.

o Also consider viral infections (see Chapter 9).

7.5 Duration of Antibiotic Treatment and Discontinuation Criteria

The optimal duration of antibiotic treatment in NF is often debated and must be individualised [1, 3].

- **If an infectious site is identified and a pathogen documented:** The duration is that recommended for treating this specific infection (e.g. 714

days for BGN bacteraemia, 5-7 days for uncomplicated pyelonephritis, etc.).

- **If fever resolved, patient stable, but focus not identified and cultures negative:**

  ◦ Antibiotic therapy is generally continued **until the patient is apyretic for at least 48 hours AND the PNN count is > 0.5 G/L (500/mm^3) and rising.**

  ◦ If the patient is low risk and treated as an outpatient, a fixed duration of 5-7 days may be considered if there is rapid resolution of symptoms and neutropenia.

- **If fever persists but the patient is stable and PNN are recovering (>0.5 G/L):**

  ◦ If no outbreak is identified and cultures remain negative, discontinuation of antibiotics may be discussed after 4-5 days of apyrexia, even if fever has persisted during neutropenia. This situation requires careful clinical judgement.

- **Persistent neutropenia:** If neutropenia persists beyond 7-10 days and the patient is apyretic and stable, the duration of antibiotic therapy is more controversial. Some continue until the neutropenia subsides, while others may stop earlier if no infection is documented.
- The use of biomarkers such as procalcitonin (monitoring its kinetics) can help guide the decision to stop antibiotics (PCT- guided discontinuation), but this needs to be validated in institutional protocols [5].

Conclusion

Systematic reassessment of the febrile neutropenic patient at H48-H72 is a fundamental step in optimising antibiotic management. Depending on the clinical course and microbiological results, treatment can be adapted, de-escalated where possible, or intensified in the event of non-response or worsening. Managing the different clinical scenarios requires sharp clinical judgement and a good knowledge of treatment options. The duration of antibiotic treatment must be individualised, with the aim of treating the infection effectively while minimising the risks associated with prolonged antibiotic therapy. The management of fungal and viral infections, which can occur in the setting of persistent fever, will be discussed in subsequent chapters.

References

1. Freifeld AG, Bow EJ, Sepkowitz KA, et al. Clinical practice guideline for the use of antimicrobial agents in neutropenic patients with cancer: 2010 update by the Infectious Diseases Society of America. Clin Infect Dis. 2011;52(4):e56-e93.
2. Leibovici L, Paul M, Poznanski O, et al. Monotherapy versus beta-

lactamaminoglycoside combination treatment for gram-negative bacteremia: a prospective, observational study. Antimicrob Agents Chemother. 2004;48(3):1127-1133.

3. Klastersky J, de Naurois J, Rolston K, et al. Management of febrile neutropaenia: ESMO Clinical Practice Guidelines. Ann Oncol. 2016;27(suppl 5):v111-v118.

4. Taplitz RA, Kennedy EB, Bow EJ, et al. Outpatient Management of Febrile Neutropenia in Adults Treated for Malignancy: American Society of Clinical Oncology and Infectious Diseases Society of America Clinical Practice Guideline Update. J Clin Oncol. 2018;36(14):1443-1453.

5. Schuetz P, Briel M, Christ-Crain M, et al. Procalcitonin to guide initiation and duration of antibiotic treatment in respiratory infections: a patient data meta-analysis. Clin Infect Dis. 2012;55(5):651-662.

6. Masterton RG. Antibiotic de-escalation. Crit Care Clin. 2011;27(1):149-162.

Chapter 8: Management of Invasive Fungal Infections (IFIs) in the Neutropenic Febrile Patient

Introduction

Invasive fungal infections (IFIs) represent a formidable and often difficult-to-diagnose complication in cancer patients with prolonged or profound febrile neutropenia. Despite advances in diagnostic tools and therapeutic options, IFI remains associated with significant morbidity and mortality [1, 2]. The pathogens most frequently implicated are yeasts of the *Candida* genus and moulds, mainly *Aspergillus spp.* Strong clinical suspicion, a diagnostic approach combining biological markers, imaging and sometimes invasive sampling, and an appropriate antifungal treatment strategy (empirical, preemptive or curative) are crucial to improving the prognosis [3]. This chapter describes the risk factors for IFI, the clinical situations in which IFI should be suspected, diagnostic tools, the different therapeutic approaches and the main classes of antifungal agents.

8.1 Risk factors for Invasive Fungal Infection (IFI) in neutropenic patients

Identification of patients at high risk of IFI is essential to guide surveillance, diagnosis and prophylactic or pre-emptive strategies. The main risk factors include [1, 2, 4] :

- Characteristics of Neutropenia:

○ **Depth:** PNN < 0.1 G/L (profound neutropenia).

○ **Duration:** severe neutropenia (PNN < 0.5 G/L) prolonged, typically > 7-10 days. Risk increases exponentially with duration of neutropenia.

- **Type of underlying pathology :**

○ **Malignant haemopathies:** acute leukaemias (myeloid and lymphoblastic) in induction or consolidation phase, high-risk myelodysplastic syndromes, bone marrow aplasia.

○ **Haematopoietic stem cell transplantation (HSCT):** Mainly allogeneic, due to the immunosuppression induced to prevent graft-versus-host disease (GVHD).

- **Immunosuppressive treatments :**

○ **High dose and/or prolonged corticosteroid therapy** (e.g. >0.3 mg/kg/d prednisone equivalent for >3 weeks).

○ Other immunosuppressants (e.g. ciclosporin, mycophenolate mofetil, alemtuzumab).

- **Other factors :**

○ Previous or current colonisation by yeasts or moulds.

Altered mucosal barriers (severe mucositis).

o Presence of central venous catheters (especially for candidemia).
o Prolonged broad-spectrum antibiotic therapy (favouring dysbiosis and yeast selection).
o Severe malnutrition.
o Hospital environment (construction work, air contamination by Aspergillus spores).
o Certain solid tumours with intensive treatment and prolonged neutropenia.

Table 8.1: Main risk factors for Invasive Fungal Infection (IFI) in neutropenic patients based on ECIL/ESCMID/IDSA recommendations [1, 2, 4]].

Category	Major Factors	Relative risk
Neutropenia	- PNN <0.1 G/L	+++
	- Duration >7-10 days	
Pathology	- Acute leukaemia	+++
	- Allogeneic HSC transplantation	
Treatment	- Corticoids >3 weeks	++
	- Heavy immunosuppressive drugs	
Other	- Central catheters	+
	• Severe mucositis	
	• Prolonged antibiotics	

8.2 When to suspect IFI Clinical and Radiological Warning Signs

Suspicion of IFI should be raised in high-risk patients, particularly in certain clinical situations [1, 3, 5]:

- **Persistent fever despite broad-spectrum antibiotic therapy:** This is the most common scenario. A fever that persists or recurs after 4 to 7 days of well-administered empirical antibiotic therapy in a patient who remains neutropenic should raise the possibility of an IFI, in particular invasive aspergillosis or disseminated candidiasis.
- **Appearance of new lung infiltrates on chest imaging:**

o In a febrile neutropenic patient, any new pulmonary radiological abnormality (nodule, consolidation, ground-glass infiltrate) should raise suspicion of a fungal origin, in particular invasive pulmonary aspergillosis (IPA).

o Specific radiological signs on chest CT, such as the "halo sign" (an area of ground-glass surrounding a dense nodule, early in the disease) or the " gas crescent sign" (an area of aerated lysis around the periphery of a necrotic nodule, later in the disease), are suggestive of IPA but are inconsistent and not pathognomonic [6].

- **Other suggestive clinical signs (depending on location):**
  - **Invasive sinusitis:** Facial pain, nasal obstruction, purulent or bloody discharge, sometimes necrosis of the palate or nasal cavities.
  - **Skin involvement:** nodular, papular or pustular lesions, sometimes with a necrotic centre (ecthyma gangrenosum, which may also be bacterial but should be considered for Fusarium or Mucorales).
  - **Disseminated candidiasis with deep organ involvement:** hepatosplenic (multiple lesions on imaging), ocular (chorioretinitis, endophthalmitis), renal, cerebral.
  - **Candida ffisophagitis**: Odynophagia, dysphagia.
  - Neurological symptoms if cerebral involvement (fungal abscess, meningitis).

8.3 Diagnosis of IFI: A Combined Approach

The definitive diagnosis of an IFI is based on the detection of the fungus in a normally sterile site (by direct examination and/or culture of a biopsy or deep sample). However, these samples are often difficult to obtain or invasive in fragile patients. Diagnosis is therefore frequently based on a combination of clinical, imaging and non-specific or specific biological markers [1, 2, 3, 5]. The EORTC/MSG (European Organization for Research and Treatment of Cancer / Mycoses Study Group) criteria are used to classify IFIs as "proven", "probable" or "possible" [4].

- 8.3.1 Biological Fungal Serological markers :

- **Galactomannan (GM) antigen:**
  - Component of the wall of *Aspergillus spp.* (and other moulds). Detectable in serum and BAL.
  - A threshold of positivity (index >0.5 or >1.0 depending on the tests and laboratories) in serum (at least two consecutive positive samples) or a higher threshold in BAL is suggestive of invasive aspergillosis (mycological criterion for a probable IFI).
  - Variable sensitivity and specificity. False positives (certain antibiotics, diet, other fungi) and false negatives (localised forms, early antifungal treatment) possible [1, 5].
- **(1 >3)-[M)-Gliicane (BDG) :**
  - Wall component of most pathogenic fungi (except Mucorales and Cryptococcus). Non-specific IFI marker.
  - A high level in the serum is an argument for an IFI, but does not identify the fungus.
  - False positives (dialysis, IV immunoglobulins, certain bacteria) and false negatives possible [1, 5].

○ **Fungal PCR (Polymerase Chain Reaction):** Detection of fungal DNA (e.g. *Aspergillus* PCR, *Candida* PCR, Panfungal PCR) in blood, BAL or other biological fluids. Their place in the diagnostic algorithm is still being validated and standardised, but they are increasingly used [1, 5].

- **8.3.2 Imaging (see section 8.2) :**

○ **High-resolution chest CT** is the gold standard for suspicion of lung involvement. Repeat examinations may be necessary to monitor the evolution of lesions.

○ Sinus CT is indicated if invasive sinusitis is suspected.

○ Ultrasound or abdominal CT/MRI if hepato-splenic candidiasis is suspected.

○ Cerebral MRI if neurological damage is suspected.

- **8.3.3 Directed microbiological sampling and histopathological examination :**

○ **Bronchoalveolar lavage (BAL) by bronchial fibroscopy:** Indicated if pulmonary infiltrates are accessible. Allows testing for GM, BDG, fungal PCR, direct examination (Gram stain, Giemsa, calcofluor) and culture for fungi.

○ **Transbronchial (BTB) or Percutaneous Biopsies:** If accessible nodular lung lesion and non-contributory BAL. Allows histopathological examination (looking for hyphae invading the tissues) and cultures.

○ **Blood cultures on specific media (e.g. Myco/F Lytic):** Useful for diagnosing candidaemia, but not very sensitive for moulds.

○ **Puncture/biopsy of other suspect sites** (skin, sinus, liver, etc.).

8.4 Antifungal treatment: Empirical, Preemptive or Curative strategies

The antifungal treatment strategy depends on the level of suspicion and diagnostic certainty, as well as the patient's risk [1, 3, 5].

- 8.4.1 Empirical antifungal treatment :

○ **Definition:** Initiation of antifungal treatment in a high-risk neutropenic patient presenting with persistent fever (>4-7 days) despite well-administered broad-spectrum antibiotics, and in whom IFI is suspected but not proven.

○ **Objective: To** treat occult IFI early and reduce mortality.

○ **Recommended molecules :**

■ **Caspofungin (echinocandin)** or other echinocandins (micafungin, anidulafungin): Good activity on *Candida spp.* (including fluconazole-resistant) and moderate activity on *Aspergillus spp*. Well tolerated.

■ **Liposomal amphotericin B (L-AMB) :** Broad spectrum (Candida, Aspergillus, Mucorales). More toxic (nephrotoxicity, electrolyte disorders).

■ **Voriconazole (azole):** Very good activity on *Aspergillus spp.* and most

Candida spp. (except *C. krusei* and some *C. glabrata*). Numerous drug interactions, serum levels sometimes need to be monitored.

■ The choice depends on the desired spectrum (anti-Aspergillus coverage required?), local epidemiology, patient co-morbidities and drug interactions.

- **8.4.2 Pre-emptive (or Biomarker-Guided) Antifungal Therapy :**

o **Definition:** Initiation of antifungal treatment in a high-risk neutropenic patient who is asymptomatic or paucisymptomatic, but has positive IFI markers (e.g. positive serum GM on two occasions, chest CT scan with suggestive images) without a definite diagnosis.

o **Objective:** Treat IFI at a very early stage to improve prognosis, while avoiding systematic empirical treatment.

o **Molecules:** Generally those used for curative treatment (voriconazole or L-AMB if aspergillosis is suspected, echinocandin if candidiasis is suspected).

- **8.4.3 Curative (or Targeted) Antifungal Treatment :**

o **Definition:** Treatment of proven (positive culture from a sterile site, histology) or probable (combination of host factors, clinical/radiological signs, and mycological criteria) IFI.

o **Choice of compound:** Depends on the fungus identified and its sensitivity (if available).

■ **Invasive candidiasis :**

■ **Echinocandin (caspofungin, micafungin, anidulafungin)** as first-line treatment.

■ Oral replacement with fluconazole (if susceptible strain) or voriconazole after clinical stabilisation and negative blood cultures.

■ Alternatively, liposomal amphotericin B.

■ **Invasive aspergillosis:**

■ **Voriconazole** (PO or IV) is the treatment of choice.

■ **Isavuconazole** (PO or IV) is a first-line alternative.

■ **Liposomal amphotericin B** as a second-line treatment or if azoles are contraindicated.

■ Combinations of antifungal agents (e.g. voriconazole + echinocandin) in severe or refractory forms (limited level of evidence).

■ **Mucormycosis (rare but very aggressive) :**

■ **High-dose liposomal amphotericin B** as first-line treatment.

■ Posaconazole or isavuconazole as consolidation or salvage treatment.

■ Surgical debridement often necessary.

■

Table 8.2: Antifungal strategies for febrile neutropenia

Strategy	Indications	1st line drugs	Alternatives	Duration
Empirical	Fever >4-7 days on broad-spectrum ATBs	Caspofungin (70mg D1 then 50mg/d IV)	L-AMB (3mg/kg/d IV)	Until NF resolution
Preemptive	Positive markers (GM+/ß-D- glucan+) or suggestive CT lesions	Voriconazole (6mg/kg x2 D1 then 4mg/kg x2 IV/PO)	Isavuconazole (200mg x3d then 200mg/d)	Minimum 14 days after negativation
Curative	IFI proven/probable	Depending on pathogen (see below)		4-6 weeks

Figure 8.1: Curative antifungal agents by pathogen

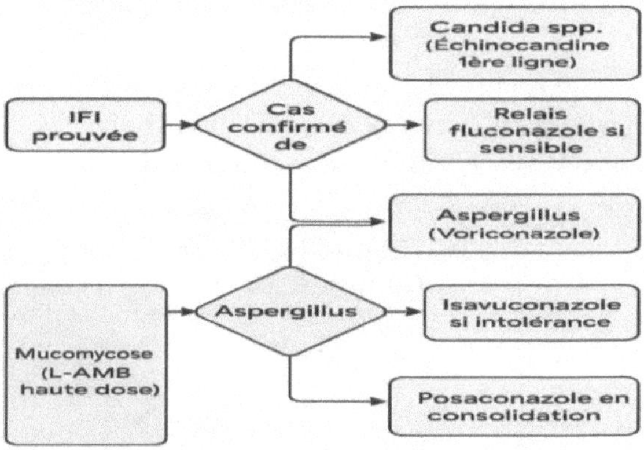

Table 8. 3: Characteristics of the main antifungal classes

Class	Drugs	Spectrum	Major toxicity	Monitoring
Echinocaine	Caspofungin/Micafungin	Candida spp. (including resistant)	Low toxicity	Alkaline phosphatases
Azoles	Voriconazole	Sensitive Aspergillus/Candida	Hepatic/neuro/QQT	Serum levels (Cmin 1-5mg/L)
Polyenes	L-AMB	Broad spectrum (except Scedosporium)	Nephro/electrolytic	Creatinine/K+/Mg++

8.5 Duration of antifungal treatment

The duration of antifungal treatment is often prolonged and depends on several factors [1, 3, 5] :

- The type of IFI and the pathogen involved.
- The severity of infection and extent of lesions.
- The clinical, radiological and mycological response to treatment.
- The patient's immune status and recovery from neutropenia.
- **Candidaemia:** At least 14 days after the first negative blood culture AND resolution of signs and symptoms of infection.
- **Invasive aspergillosis**: Prolonged treatment, often for several weeks to months (at least 6-12 weeks), until significant resolution or stabilisation of radiological lesions and depending on immunosuppression. Maintenance

treatment may be necessary if immunosuppression persists.

•

- The decision to stop antifungal treatment must be individualised and taken in consultation with specialists (infectiologist, haematologist/oncologist).

Figure 8.2: Decision-making tree for the management of IFIs

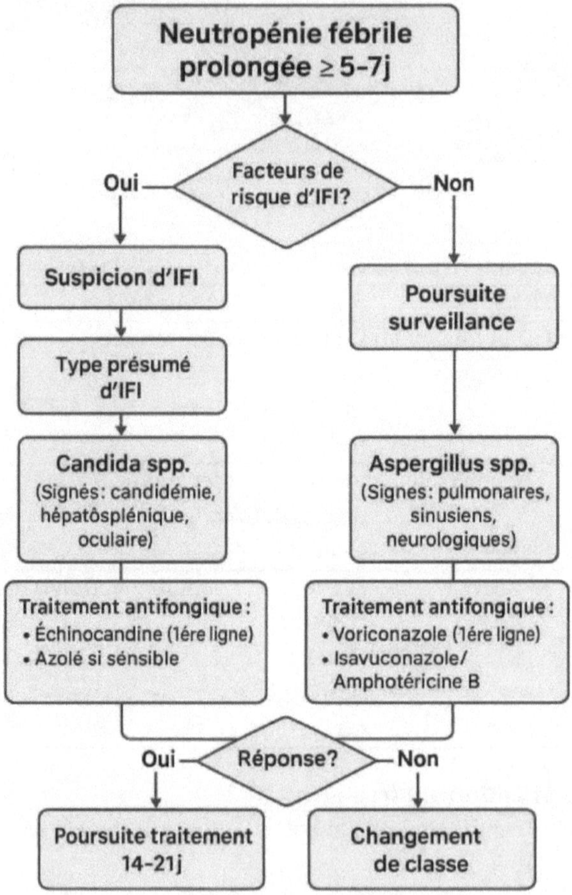

Conclusion

Invasive fungal infections are a serious threat to febrile neutropenic patients, particularly those with profound and prolonged neutropenia or other risk factors. High clinical suspicion in cases of unexplained persistent fever or new pulmonary signs is crucial. Diagnosis is based on a combination of clinical, radiological and fungal biomarkers, with histopathological or culture confirmation being the gold standard but not always feasible. The therapeutic strategy (empirical, preemptive or curative) and the choice of antifungal agent depend on the clinical context, the suspected or identified pathogen, and the patient's characteristics. Multidisciplinary management and careful monitoring are essential to optimise the prognosis of these serious infections.

References

1. Patterson TF, Thompson GR 3rd, Denning DW, et al. Practice Guidelines for the Diagnosis and Management of Aspergillosis: 2016 Update by the Infectious Diseases Society of America. Clin Infect Dis. 2016;63(4):e1- e60.
2. Pappas PG, Kauffman CA, Andes DR, et al. Clinical Practice Guideline for the Management of Candidiasis: 2016 Update by the Infectious Diseases Society of America. Clin Infect Dis. 2016;62(4):e1-e50.
3. Freifeld AG, Bow EJ, Sepkowitz KA, et al. Clinical practice guideline for the use of antimicrobial agents in neutropenic patients with cancer: 2010 update by the Infectious Diseases Society of America. Clin Infect Dis. 2011;52(4):e56-e93.
4. De Pauw B, Walsh TJ, Donnelly JP, et al. Revised definitions of invasive fungal disease from the European Organization for Research and Treatment of Cancer/Invasive Fungal Infections Cooperative Group and the National Institute of Allergy and Infectious Diseases Mycoses Study Group (EORTC/MSG) Consensus Group. Clin Infect Dis. 2008;46(12):1813- 1821.
5. Maertens JA, Girmenia C, Brüggemann RJ, et al. European Conference on Infections in Leukaemia (ECIL-6) guidelines for the treatment of invasive fungal diseases (aspergillosis, mucormycosis and cryptococcosis) in adult patients with haematological malignancies and CML. Haematologica. 2018;103(3)
6. Caillot D, Couaillier JF, Bernard A, et al. Increasing volume and enhancing halo sign on early computed tomography predict unfavorable outcome in invasive pulmonary aspergillosis. J Clin Oncol. 2001 Mar 1;19(5):1534- 1541.

Chapter 9: Management of Viral Infections in the Febrile Neutropenic Patient

Introduction

Although bacterial and fungal infections are the major concerns in febrile neutropenia (NF), viral infections are also a significant cause of morbidity and sometimes mortality in immunocompromised cancer patients. These infections may result from the reactivation of latent viruses (particularly those of the Herpes group) or from primary infection with community-acquired viruses, especially respiratory viruses [1, 2]. The clinical presentation of viral infections can be atypical in neutropenic patients, and their diagnosis is often based on molecular biology techniques (PCR). Early recognition and targeted antiviral treatment, where available, are essential to limit the impact of these infections [3]. This chapter looks at the main viral infections encountered in this context, their manifestations, diagnosis and management.

9.1 Reactivation of Herpes group viruses (Herpesviridae)

Herpes group viruses (Herpes Simplex Virus type 1 and 2 - HSV-1/2, Varicella-Zoster Virus - VZV, Cytomegalovirus - CMV, Epstein-Barr Virus - EBV) are characterised by their ability to establish latency in the body after primary infection, with a risk of reactivation in the event of immunosuppression.

. 9.1.1 Herpes Simplex Virus (HSV-1 and HSV-2)

- **Epidemiology and risk factors:** HSV reactivation is common in HIV-positive patients receiving intensive chemotherapy, HSC transplants or corticosteroids. Severe mucositis is a major risk factor for oral lesions [4].
- **Clinical presentation :**
  - Oral-facial herpes (HSV-1) Vesicular lesions

on the lips, buccal mucosa, tongue and palate. In neutropenic patients, vesicles may be absent or atypical, presenting as extensive and very painful necrotic ulcerations, difficult to distinguish from pure mucositis.

  - Genital herpes (mainly HSV-2): Similar lesions on external genitalia, perineum.
  - More rarely: herpetic sopliagitis (odynophagia, dysphagia), herpetic keratitis, herpetic meningoencephalitis, disseminated herpes (potentially fatal).
- **Diagnosis :**
  - Swabbing of lesions for HSV PCR (highly sensitive and specific).
  - Tzanck cytodiagnostic examination (for multinucleated giant cells, less sensitive).

■ Biopsy with immunohistochemistry if lesions are atypical.

○ **Treatment:**

■ Aciclovir: Intravenous (5-10 mg/kg every 8 hours) for severe, widespread or disseminated forms. Oral relay with valaciclovir or famciclovir after improvement.

■ Topical treatment (aciclovir cream) not very effective on extensive mucosal lesions.

■ Treatment of aciclovir-resistant strains (rare): foscarnet, cidofovir.

○ **Prophylaxis:** Aciclovir or oral valaciclovir in HSV-positive patients at high risk of reactivation (e.g. induction of acute leukaemia, HSC transplant, expected severe mucositis) [1, 3].

- 9.1.2 Varicella-Zoster Virus (VZV)

○ **Epidemiology and risk factors:** VZV reactivation (herpes zoster) is common in immunocompromised patients, particularly those with haematological malignancies or on corticosteroid therapy.

○ **Clinical presentation :**

■ Localized shingles: Painful, unilateral, vesicular eruption following a dermatome. May be preceded by neuropathic pain.

■ Disseminated (varicella-like) or visceral (pulmonary, hepatic, neurological) shingles: Severe, potentially lethal forms, more common in highly immunocompromised patients.

Diagnosis :

■ Mainly clinical if typical.

■ VZV PCR on vesicular fluid or skin biopsy.

■ If visceral involvement: VZV PCR on BAL, CSF, blood.

○ **Treatment:**

■ Aciclovir IV (10 mg/kg every 8 hours) for all shingles in an immunocompromised patient, especially if extensive, ophthalmic, or if visceral involvement. Oral relay with valaciclovir or famciclovir.

■ Appropriate analgesic treatment.

○ **Prophylaxis:** Aciclovir or oral valaciclovir in high-risk patients (e.g. HSC transplants, treatment with alemtuzumab or proteasome inhibitors) [1, 3]. VZV vaccination (live attenuated vaccine) is contraindicated in actively immunocompromised patients; recombinant inactivated vaccine (Shingrix®) may be discussed prior to immunosuppression or at a later stage.

- 9.1.3 Cytomegalovirus (CMV)

○ **Epidemiology and risk factors:** CMV reactivation is a major complication in HSC allograft recipients and solid organ transplant recipients. It can also occur in other highly immunocompromised patients (e.g. acute leukaemia undergoing intensive chemotherapy, high-dose corticosteroid therapy).

○ **Clinical presentation:** Often asymptomatic (CMV viremia detected by PCR). If CMV disease :

■ Flu-like syndrome (fever, myalgias, asthenia).

■ CMV interstitial lung disease (dyspnoea, cough, hypoxia).

■ CMV colitis (diarrhoea, abdominal pain, rectal discharge).

■ Hepatitis, retinitis (especially if CD4 is low), encephalitis.

○ **Diagnosis :**

■ Quantitative CMV PCR in blood (CMV viral load): Key tool for diagnosis and monitoring of reactivation/infection.

■ CMV PCR on BAL, digestive biopsies, CSF.

■ Histology (search for "owl's eye" viral inclusions) on biopsies.

○ **Treatment (preemptive or curative strategy):**

■ Ganciclovir IV or its oral prodrug valganciclovir are the treatments of choice.

■ Foscarnet or cidofovir in case of resistance or intolerance.

○ **Prophylaxis/pre-emptive treatment:** In high-risk patients (allograft recipients), regular monitoring of CMV viral load and initiation of pre-emptive treatment (valganciclovir, letermovir) if viremia is significant [1, 3, 5].

- 9.1.4 Epstein-Barr Virus (EBV)

○ EBV reactivation in immunocompromised patients may be associated with post-transplant lymphoproliferative disorders (PTLD) or other EBV-related lymphoproliferative disorders. It is less frequently a direct cause of acute febrile syndrome in NF outside these contexts.

Diagnosis: EBV PCR in blood, tissue biopsies.

Treatment: Reduction in immunosuppression if possible, rituximab, chemotherapy (for PTLD). Specific antivirals have limited efficacy.

9.2 Community-acquired respiratory viruses

Respiratory viral infections are common and may be particularly severe in neutropenic patients, with a risk of pneumonitis and respiratory distress.

• **9.2.1 Influenza viruses (Influenza A and B)**

○ **Clinical presentation:** Sudden onset of fever, cough, myalgias, headache, asthenia. May be complicated by primary viral pneumonitis or bacterial superinfection.

Diagnosis: PCR on nasopharyngeal swab.

○ **Treatment:** Neuraminidase inhibitors (oseltamivir, zanamivir, peramivir) or baloxavir, to be started as early as possible (<48 hours ideally, but benefits even if delayed in immunocompromised patients) [1, 3, 6].

- **Prevention:** Annual vaccination of all cancer patients and their families. Prophylaxis with oseltamivir during epidemics in the case of high-risk contacts or unvaccinated patients.

- **9.2.2 Respiratory Syncytial Virus (RSV)**

- **Clinical presentation:** nasopharyngitis, cough, dyspnoea, wheezing. May progress to bronchiolitis or severe pneumonitis, especially in highly immunocompromised patients (allograft recipients).

Diagnosis: PCR on nasopharyngeal swab.

- **Treatment:** Ribavirin (aerosol or IV) discussed for severe forms in high-risk patients (controversial efficacy, toxicity) [1, 3]. Palivizumab for prophylaxis in certain at-risk children (not applicable to neutropenic adults). Nirsevimab is a new monoclonal antibody for prophylaxis in infants.

- **9.2.3 Other respiratory viruses :**

- Human metapneumovirus (hMPV), Parainfluenza virus (PIV), Rhinovirus, Adenovirus, Bocavirus, non-SARS-CoV-2 Coronavirus: Can cause upper and lower airway infections of varying severity [7, 8].
- **Diagnosis:** multiplex PCR on nasopharyngeal swabs.
- **Treatment:** Mostly symptomatic. Cidofovir may be discussed for disseminated or severe adenovirus infections.

. 9.2.4 SARS-CoV-2 (COVID-19)

- **Clinical presentation:** Broad spectrum, from asymptomatic infection to severe hypoxaemic pneumonitis and ARDS. Cancer patients, especially those on active treatment or with co-morbidities, are at risk of severe forms [9].
- **Diagnosis:** PCR on nasopharyngeal swab or low respiratory specimen. Chest CT scan.
- **Treatment (evolves rapidly, refer to updated recommendations):**

▪ Antivirals (e.g. nirmatrelvir/ritonavir (Paxlovid®), remdesivir) in patients at risk of progression to a severe form, to be initiated early.

▪ Immunomodulators (dexamethasone, tocilizumab, baricitinib) for hypoxaemic forms.

▪ Neutralising monoclonal antibodies (variable efficacy depending on the variant).

- **Prevention:** Vaccination (primary and booster), barrier measures.

9.3 General measures and prevention of viral infections

- Standard Precautions and Hygiene Measures: Wash hands, wear a mask during respiratory viral epidemics, avoid contact with sick people.
- Vaccinations: Update vaccination schedule before starting immunosuppressive treatments if possible (annual influenza, pneumococcus,

COVID-19). Live attenuated vaccines (MMR, VZV, yellow fever) are generally contraindicated during immunosuppression.

• Targeted antiviral prophylaxis (see specific sections on HSV, VZV, CMV, influenza) in high-risk patients.

• Management of the hospital environment to limit nosocomial transmission of respiratory viruses.

Conclusion

Viral infections, whether reactivations of latent Herpes viruses or infections by community-acquired respiratory viruses, account for a significant proportion of infectious complications in febrile neutropenic patients. Their clinical presentation can be atypical and their impact potentially severe, particularly for CMV, disseminated VZV, influenza, RSV or SARS-CoV-2 in profoundly immunocompromised patients. Diagnosis is essentially based on PCR techniques. Specific antiviral treatments are available for several of these infections, and early initiation is often the key to success. Prophylaxis and vaccination strategies, where possible, play a crucial role in preventing these viral infections. Constant vigilance and a proactive diagnostic approach are needed to optimise the management of these patients.

References

1. Freifeld AG, Bow EJ, Sepkowitz KA, et al. Clinical practice guideline for the use of antimicrobial agents in neutropenic patients with cancer: 2010 update by the Infectious Diseases Society of America. Clin Infect Dis. 2011;52(4):e56-e93.

2. Styczynski J, van der Velden W, Fox CP, et al. Management of Epstein-Barr virus infections and post-transplant lymphoproliferative disorders in patients after allogeneic hematopoietic stem cell transplantation: Sixth European Conference on Infections in Leukemia (ECIL-6) guidelines. Haematologica. 2016;101(7):803-811.

3. Tomblyn M, Chiller T, Einsele H, et al. Guidelines for preventing infectious complications among hematopoietic cell transplantation recipients: a global perspective. Biol Blood Marrow Transplant. 2009;15(10):1143-1238.

4. Glenister H, Coyle P, Gleadall A, et al. Herpes simplex virus infections in immunocompromised patients. Herpes. 2005;12(1):10-14.

5. Ljungman P, de la Camara R, Robin C, et al. Guidelines for the management of cytomegalovirus infection in patients with haematological malignancies and after stem cell transplantation from the 2017 European Conference on Infections in Leukaemia (ECIL 7). Lancet Infect Dis. 2019;19(8):e260-e272.

6. Uyeki TM, Bernstein HH, Bradley JS, et al. Clinical Practice Guidelines by the Infectious Diseases Society of America: 2018 Update on Diagnosis, Treatment, Chemoprophylaxis, and Institutional Outbreak Management of Seasonal Influenza. Clin Infect Dis. 2019;68(6):e1-e47.
7. Hirsch HH, Martino R, Ward KN, et al. Fourth European Conference on Infections in Leukaemia (ECIL-4): guidelines for diagnosis and treatment of human respiratory syncytial virus, parainfluenza virus, metapneumovirus, rhinovirus, and coronavirus. Clin Infect Dis. 2013;56(2):258-266.
8. Chemaly RF, Shah DP, Boeckh MJ. Management of respiratory viral infections in hematopoietic cell transplant recipients and patients with hematologic malignancies. Clin Infect Dis. 2014;59 Suppl 5:S344-S351.
9. Vijenthira A, Gong IY, Fox TA, et al. Outcomes of patients with hematologic malignancies and COVID-19: a systematic review and metaanalysis of 3377 patients. Blood. 2020;136(25):2881-2892.

Chapter 10: Management of Non-Infectious Complications and Symptoms
Associated with Febrile Neutropenia

Introduction

The management of febrile neutropenia (NF) is not limited to the treatment of the underlying infection. Neutropenic patients, often debilitated by their cancer and anti-cancer treatments, frequently present with a constellation of non-infectious complications and associated symptoms that can be just as debilitating as the infection itself. Mucositis, non-infectious diarrhoea, pain, anxiety, sleep disturbance and undernutrition are common problems that significantly impair quality of life, can compromise adherence to treatment and prolong hospitalisation [1, 2]. A proactive approach, incorporating optimised supportive care, is therefore essential for comprehensive and humane patient management. This chapter describes the management of these complications and frequently encountered symptoms.

10.1 Management of Oral and Digestive Mucositis

Mucositis, an inflammation of the mucous membranes, is a frequent and painful complication of chemotherapy and radiotherapy. It can affect the entire digestive tract, from the mouth to the anus.

- **10.1.1 Pathophysiology and risk factors**

  - Direct toxicity of cytotoxic agents on rapidly renewing epithelial cells [3].
  - Release of pro-inflammatory cytokines.
  - Alteration of the local microbiota.
  - Risk factors: type of chemotherapy (e.g. 5-FU, methotrexate, anthracyclines, etoposide), dose, concomitant radiotherapy (especially ENT or pelvic), poor oral hygiene, smoking, alcoholism.

- **10.1.2 Clinical presentation and grading**

Oral mucositis: erythema, swelling, burning, pain, mouth ulcers, pseudomembranes, bleeding, dysphagia, dysgeusia.

  - **Digestive mucosa (esophagitis, enteritis, non-infectious colitis):** Odynophagia, dysphagia, abdominal pain, diarrhoea, nausea, vomiting, rectal bleeding.
  - **Grading (CTCAE v5.0 "Oral mucositis", "ffisophagitis", "Enteritis", etc.) [4]:** Based on symptoms, appearance of lesions, and impact on diet and ADLs.

- **10.1.3 Prevention**

  - **Rigorous oral hygiene:** gentle brushing after each meal, non-alcoholic mouthwashes (e.g. sodium bicarbonate, saline solution).
  - Dental examination and preventive care before chemotherapy/radiotherapy.

○ Oral cryotherapy (sucking on ice cubes) during the infusion of certain agents (e.g. 5-FU, melphalan) [5].

○ Palifermin (keratinocyte growth factor): indicated for the prevention of severe mucositis in patients receiving high-dose chemotherapy prior to HSC autotransplantation for haematological malignancies [1, 2].

- **10.1.4 Treatment**

○ **Symptomatic treatment:**

■ **Pain:** Analgesics adapted to the intensity (paracetamol, weak to strong opioids). Topical anaesthetic solutions (viscous lidocaine, "magic" solutions with antacid/antihistamine/anaesthetic - caution with systemic absorption).

■ **Hygiene:** Mild antiseptic mouthwashes should be continued.

■ **Hydration and nutrition:** Prefer soft, cold, non-irritating foods. Nutritional support (enteral or parenteral) if severe mucositis prevents feeding.

○ **Specific treatments (variable efficacy, often limited):**

■ Growth factors (G-CSF, GM-CSF) as mouthwashes (off-label use).

■ Low-energy laser therapy (LLLT): promising results in some studies for prevention and treatment [6].

■ Sucralfate, amifostine (effectiveness debated).

○ Exclude and treat superinfection (candidiasis, herpes).

Table

at u 10.1: Treatment strategies by grade of mucositis

Grade	Clinical signs	Treatment	Monitoring
1	Erythema without ulceration	Strict hygiene + mouthwash (bicarbonate/salt)	Daily assessment
2	Ulcers <1cm, feeding possible	Analgesics (paracetamol + tramadol) + anaesthetic gel	Nutritional adjustment
3	Ulcers confluent, dysphagia	Morphine + nutrition enteral/probe + photobiomodulation	Prevention of complications
4	Necrosis/haemorrhage	Hospital admission + intensive care + empirical antibiotic therapy	Haemodynamic monitoring

Figure 10.1: Grading and management of mucositis

(Adapted from WHO and NCI CTCAE v5.0 scales)

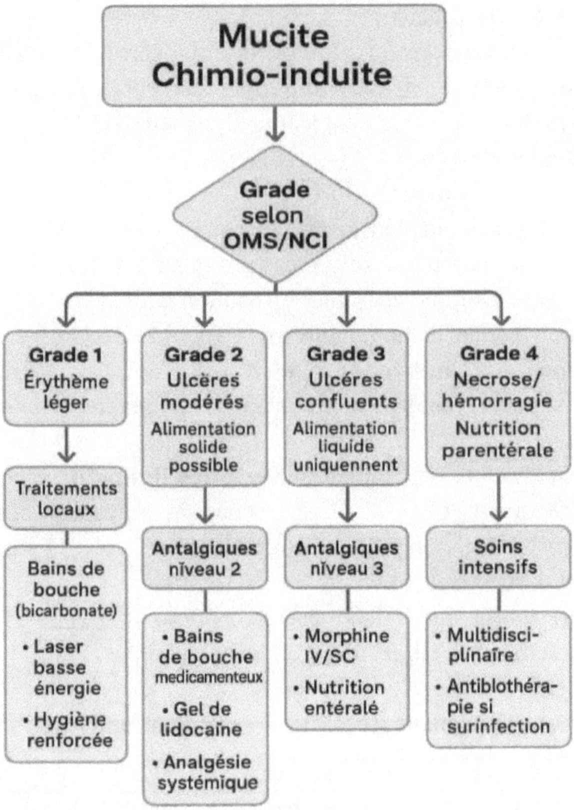

10.2 Management of non-infectious diarrhoea

Diarrhoea in neutropenic patients may be infectious (see Chapter 5) or non-infectious (related to chemotherapy, radiotherapy or digestive mucositis).

- **10.2.1 Non-infectious causes of diarrhoea**

◦ Direct toxicity of chemotherapy on the intestinal mucosa (e.g. irinotecan, 5-FU, tyrosine kinase inhibitors).

◦ Radiation enteritis (if pelvic or abdominal irradiation).

◦ Malabsorption (e.g. after digestive surgery, pancreatic insufficiency).

◦ Certain drugs (laxatives, certain antibiotics due to dysbiosis).

- **10.2.2 Assessment and differential diagnosis**

History (characteristics of diarrhoea, recent treatments, diet).

◦ Clinical examination (hydration status, abdominal signs).

◦ **Rule out an infectious cause:** stool cultures, search for *C. difficile* toxins, viral PCR (see Chapters 4 and 5).

○ Endoscopy with biopsies if severe and persistent diarrhoea with no obvious cause.

- **10.2.3 Treatment**

○ **Dietary measures:** Low-residue, lactose-free diet, avoid irritating foods. Good oral hydration (oral rehydration solutions if necessary).

○ **Transit inhibitors:**

■ Loperamide: First-line treatment. Appropriate doses (max 16 mg/d).

■ Racecadotril (intestinal enkephalinase inhibitor).

■ Octreotide (somatostatin analogue): For severe and refractory chemo-induced diarrhoea (specialist use) [1, 2].

○ Intestinal dressings (diosmectite): modest efficacy.

○ Probiotics: controversial role in neutropenic patients (theoretical risk of bacteremia/fungemia), generally not recommended in profound neutropenia [1].

○ IV fluid and electrolyte balance if dehydration.

10.3 Pain management

Pain is a frequent and disabling symptom in cancer patients, and may be exacerbated during NF episodes (mucositis, post-G-CSF bone pain, pain associated with an infectious site).

- **10.3.1 Pain assessment**

○ Systematic and repeated, using appropriate scales (Visual Analogue Scale - VAS, Numerical Scale - NRS, Simple Verbal Scale - SVS).

○ Identify the type of pain (nociceptive, neuropathic, mixed), its location, intensity and impact.

- **10.3.2 Principles of analgesic treatment (according to WHO levels)** ○ **Level 1 (mild pain) :** Paracetamol (caution if liver disease), NSAIDs (to be avoided if possible in cases of thrombocytopenia, renal failure, or risk of mucositis/digestive bleeding).

○ **Stage 2 (moderate pain or failure of Stage 1):** Weak opioids (codeine, tramadol, opium powder). Often combined with paracetamol. Beware of side effects (constipation, nausea, drowsiness).

○ **Stage 3 (severe pain or failure of Stage 2):** Strong opioids (morphine, oxycodone, hydromorphone, fentanyl). Oral route preferred, but SC or IV route if necessary (titration). Systematic prevention of constipation.

- **10.3.3 Adjuvant treatments**

○ Co-antalgesics for neuropathic pain: Gabapentin, pregabalin, tricyclic antidepressants (amitriptyline), duloxetine.

○ Corticoids (analgesic and anti-inflammatory effect, but to be used with discretion in this context).

o Muscle relaxants for contractures.

- **10.3.4 Non-pharmacological approaches**

o Relaxation, sophrology, hypnosis, TENS (transcutaneous electrical neurostimulation), physiotherapy, psychological support.

10.4 Managing anxiety and sleep disorders

The announcement of cancer, treatment, hospitalisation, fever, pain and uncertainty frequently generate significant anxiety and sleep disorders.

- **10.4.1 Assessment**

o Actively look for signs of anxiety, anguish and reactive depression.

o Assess the quality and quantity of sleep.

- **10.4.2 Treatment**

o **Psychological support:** active listening, reassurance, clear and appropriate information. Suggest follow-up by a psychologist or psychiatrist if necessary.

o **Relaxation techniques, mindfulness meditation.**

o **Sleep hygiene**: Keep to regular hours, avoid stimulants in the evening, provide a calm, dark environment.

o **Pharmacological treatments (with caution and for short periods if possible):**

■ Anxiolytics: Benzodiazepines with a short half-life (e.g. alprazolam, oxazepam) if major anxiety.

■ Hypnotics: Zolpidem, zopiclone if incapacitating insomnia.

■ Sedative antihistamines (hydroxyzine, doxylamine) may help.

■ Melatonin.

o Treat pain and other physical symptoms that may disrupt sleep.

10.5 Prevention and management of undernutrition

Undernutrition is common in cancer patients and can be exacerbated by NF, mucositis, diarrhoea, nausea/vomiting, anorexia and inflammation.

- **10.5.1 Screening and assessment of nutritional status**

o Regular weighing, calculation of BMI, assessment of recent weight loss.

o Assessment of food intake.

o Measurement of albumin and prealbumin (late markers influenced by inflammation).

- **10.5.2 Prevention and management strategies**

o **Dietary advice:** Split meals, enrich the diet (proteins, calories), adapt textures if mucositis or dysphagia.

o **Oral Nutritional Supplements (ONS)**: if intake is inadequate.

o **Enteral nutrition:** via nasogastric tube or gastrostomy if severe malnutrition and digestive tract functional but oral intake impossible or inadequate.

o **Parenteral nutrition:** if the digestive tract is non-functional (e.g. prolonged ileus, very severe digestive mucositis).
o Dietary advice and/ or assessment by a team specialising in nutrition.
o Correction of vitamin deficiencies if necessary.
o Appropriate physical activity to maintain muscle mass.

Figure 10.2: Decision-making tree for nutritional management

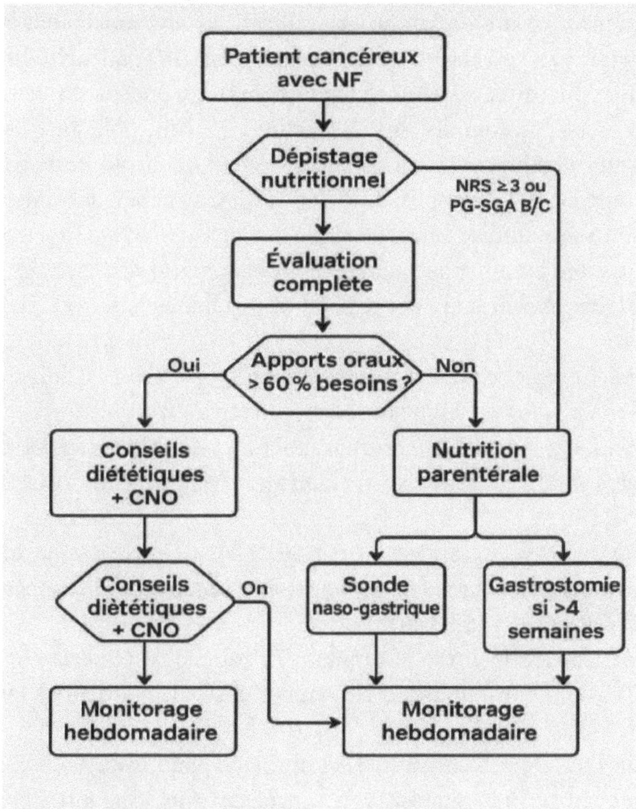

Legend :
- **NRS**: Nutritional Risk Score
- **PG-SGA**: Patient-Generated Subjective Global Assessment
- **CNO**: Oral Nutritional Supplements

10.6 Importance of Global Supportive Care

In addition to the specific aspects discussed, a global supportive care approach is essential for the well-being of the febrile neutropenic patient.

- **Communication and information:** explaining the situation, treatments, reassurance.
- **Patient comfort:** managing fever, chills, mouth care, skin care.
- **Social and family support:** Involving family and friends if the patient so

wishes.

- **Preparing for discharge from hospital**: clear instructions, organised follow-up.
- **Coordination of care** between the various people involved (doctors, nurses, dietician, psychologist, physiotherapist, social worker).

Conclusion

The management of non-infectious complications and associated symptoms is an integral part of the overall management of patients with febrile neutropenia. Mucositis, diarrhoea, pain, anxiety, sleep disturbance and malnutrition can profoundly affect quality of life, tolerance of cancer treatment and overall prognosis. Systematic assessment of these problems, a preventive approach where possible, and targeted therapeutic interventions, integrated into a multidisciplinary supportive care approach, are essential to improving patient comfort and outcomes. Listening to and empathising with patients and their families are at the heart of this humanistic approach to care.

References

1. National Comprehensive Cancer Network (NCCN). Clinical Practice Guidelines in Oncology: Palliative Care. Version 2.2021.
2. Ripamonti CI, Santini D, Maranzano E, et al. Management of cancer pain: ESMO Clinical Practice Guidelines. Ann Oncol. 2012;23 Suppl 7:vii139- vii154.
3. Lalla RV, Bowen J, Barasch A, et al. MASCC/ISOO clinical practice guidelines for the management of mucositis secondary to cancer therapy. Cancer. 2014;120(10):1453-1461.
4. National Cancer Institute. Common Terminology Criteria for Adverse Events (CTCAE) v5.0. Published November 27, 2017. Accessed January 15, 2024.
5. Peterson DE, Ohrn K, Bowen J, et al. Systematic review of ancomia for the management of oral mucositis in cancer patients. Support Care Cancer. 2013;21(1):313-321.
6. Oberoi S, Zamperlini-Netto G, Beyene J, et al. Effect of prophylactic low level laser therapy on oral mucositis: a systematic review and metaanalysis. PLoS One. 2014;9(9):e107418.

Part 4

Prevention of Febrile Neutropenia

Chapter 11: Use of Granulocyte Growth Factors (G-CSF) in the Prevention and Management of Neutropenia

Introduction

The prevention of neutropenia and its most dreaded complication, febrile neutropenia (NF), is a central objective in oncology in order to maintain the dose-intensity of chemotherapy and improve treatment tolerance. Granulocyte growth factors (G-CSF), recombinant cytokines that stimulate the production and maturation of neutrophil polynuclear cells (NPCs) by the bone marrow, play a key role in this preventive strategy [1, 2]. Their use in primary or secondary prophylaxis, based on a rigorous assessment of the risk of NF associated with chemotherapy and the patient's characteristics, is now well codified by international recommendations. This chapter details the different types of G-CSF available, their indications for prophylaxis, their (more limited) place in curative situations, the methods of administration, potential side-effects, and summarises the main recommendations of learned societies.

11.1 Types of Granulocyte Growth Factor (G-CSF)

Several recombinant forms of G-CSF are clinically available, differing mainly in their duration of action.

- **11.1.1 Short-acting G-CSF :**

  - **Filgrastim (Neupogen® and biosimilars) :** Non-glycosylated recombinant form of human G-CSF. Requires daily subcutaneous (SC) injections.
  - **Lenograstim (Granocyte® and biosimilars):** Recombinant glycosylated form of human G-CSF. Also available as daily SC injections.

- **11.1.2 Long-acting G-CSF (Pegylated) :**

These forms have a prolonged half-life due to conjugation to a polyethylene glycol (PEG) molecule, allowing single administration per chemotherapy cycle.

  - **Pegfilgrastim (Neulasta®, and its biosimilars such as Pelmeg®, Nyvepria®, Ziextenzo®, etc.):** Administered as a single SC injection per cycle, usually 24 hours after the end of chemotherapy.
  - **Lipegfilgrastim (Lonquex®):** Another pegylated form, also administered as a single SC injection per cycle.

- **G-CSF biosimilars :**

Several biosimilars of filgrastim and pegfilgrastim are now available. They have demonstrated comparable efficacy and safety to the reference products, at a potentially lower cost [3]. Their use is encouraged by the health authorities.

Table 11.1: Main G-CSFs available

Type of G-CSF	Trade name (examples)	Route of administration	Frequency of administration	Remarks
Short-term G-CSF	Filgrastim (Neupogen®, biosimilars)	Subcutaneous (SC)	Daily (1 injection/day)	Non-glycosylated form
	Lenograstim (Granocyte®, biosimilars)	Subcutaneous (SC)	Daily (1 injection/day)	Glycosylated form
Long-lasting G-CSF	Pegfilgrastim (Neulasta®, Pelmeg®, Nyvepria®, Ziextenzo®)	SC	1 injection/cycle (24h post-chemotherapy)	Pegylated, prolonged half-life
	Lipegfilgrastim (Lonquex®)	Subcutaneous (SC)	1 injection/cycle	Other pegylated form
Biosimilars	Filgrastim biosimilars (e.g. Zarzio®, Nivestim®)	SC	Daily	Comparable efficacy and safety
	Biosimilars of pegfilgrastim (e.g. Pelmeg®, Nyvepria®)	SC	1 injection/cycle	Reduced cost, use encouraged

11.2 Indications for G-CSF in primary prophylaxis

Primary prophylaxis with G-CSF consists of administering G-CSF from the first cycle of chemotherapy to prevent the occurrence of NF. Its indication is based on assessment of the risk of NF associated with the chemotherapy protocol and the patient's individual risk factors [1, 2, 4, 5].

- **11.2.1 Assessment of the risk of chemotherapy-related febrile neutropenia :**

Chemotherapy regimens are classified according to their intrinsic risk of inducing NF (see Chapter 2.2.2):

- **High risk (>20% incidence of NF): Primary prophylaxis with G-CSF systematically recommended.**
- **Intermediate risk (10-20% incidence of NF): Primary prophylaxis with G-CSF to be discussed according to the patient's individual risk factors** (see below).
- **Low risk (<10% incidence of NF): Primary prophylaxis with G-CSF generally not recommended.**

- **11.2.2 Consideration of Individual Risk Factors (for intermediate risk regimens) :**

If the chemotherapy regimen is intermediate risk, the presence of one or more of the following risk factors (described in Chapter 2.3) should prompt consideration of primary prophylaxis with G-CSF:

- Age > 65 with co-morbidities.

o Impaired general condition (ECOG PS >2).
o History of NF.
o Pre-existing neutropenia or bone marrow disease.
o Lack of social support or difficult access to care.
o Severe co-morbidities (renal, hepatic, cardiovascular).
o Expected severe mucositis.
o Active infection.

• **11.2.3 Purpose of chemotherapy (curative vs palliative) :** The indication for primary prophylaxis with G-CSF is particularly strong when the goal of treatment is curative and it is crucial to maintain the dose-intensity of chemotherapy to maximise the chance of cure (e.g. adjuvant or neoadjuvant chemotherapy, treatment of aggressive lymphomas or leukaemias) [1, 4].

Decision algorithm for primary prophylaxis with G-CSF

(Source: Adapted from ASCO 2023, ESMO 2022, NCCN 2024 [1, 4, 5])

Steps in the algorithm :

1. **Chemotherapy protocol risk assessment**:
   - o **High risk (>20% NF) Systematic primary prophylaxis with G- CSF** (Grade A).
   - o **Intermediate risk (10-20% NF) Analyse individual risk factors** (see step 2).
   - o **Low risk (<10% NF) No primary prophylaxis** (except in exceptional cases).
2. **Analysis of individual risk factors** (for intermediate regimens) :
   - o **If >1 risk factor** (list below) **Primary prophylaxis recommended** (Grade B).
   - o **If no risk factors** Strict clinical monitoring possible (Grade C).

Individual risk factors:

o Age > 65 years+ comorbidities.
o ECOG PS >2.
o History of NF or pre-existing neutropenia.
o Severe co-morbidities (renal, hepatic, etc.).
o Curative aim of treatment (e.g. adjuvant chemotherapy).

3. **Purpose of treatment** :

o **Curative** (e.g. lymphoma, adjuvant breast cancer) **Encourage prophylaxis** to maintain dose-intensity.
o **Palliative** Assess the benefit/quality of life ratio (prophylaxis if there is a high risk of complications).

11.3 Indications for G-CSF in secondary prophylaxis

Secondary prophylaxis with G-CSF consists of administering G-CSF during subsequent cycles of chemotherapy, after a patient has had an episode of NF (or prolonged neutropenia leading to a significant delay in treatment) during a previous cycle in which he or she was not receiving G- CSF as primary prophylaxis [1, 2, 4, 5].

• **Objective: To** prevent recurrence of NF and allow continuation of chemotherapy at the planned dose and schedule.

- **Indication:** Systematic after an episode of NF occurring without primary prophylaxis, if continuation of the same chemotherapy (or chemotherapy of similar risk) is planned and a reduction in dose is not desirable (especially if curative objective).

11.4 Therapeutic Use of G-CSF in Established Febrile Neutropenia

The use of G-CSF once an episode of NF has occurred ("curative" or "therapeutic" use) is a more debated subject and its indications are limited [1, 4, 5].

- **Theoretical rationale: To** accelerate the rise of PNNs and potentially reduce the duration of neutropenia and fever.
- **Clinical evidence:**
  - Randomised trials and meta-analyses have shown that the therapeutic use of G-CSF in patients with uncomplicated NF with no poor prognostic factors does not provide **any significant benefit in terms of overall mortality or length of hospitalisation**, although a modest reduction in the duration of fever and neutropenia may be observed [1, 6].
  - Its systematic use is therefore **not recommended** for all patients with NF.
- **Limited and debatable indications (to be assessed on a case-by-case basis):**
  - Patients with risk factors for serious infectious complications (e.g. PNN < 0.1 G/L, neutropenia expected >10 days, age >65 years with comorbidities, severe sepsis/septic shock, pneumonia, proven or suspected fungal infection, hypotension).
  - Failure of initial antibiotic therapy with persistent fever and profound neutropenia.
  - The decision must be individualised and taken in consultation.

11.5 Administration, duration and side effects of G-CSF

- 11.5.1 Administration :

- **Filgrastim/Lenograstim (short-acting) :**
  - Usual dose: 5 Hg/kg/day as a daily SC injection.
  - Initiation: Usually 24 to 72 hours after completion of chemotherapy. **Do not administer on the day of chemotherapy or in the 24 hours prior to chemotherapy.**
  - Duration: Continue until the PNN count has risen to a safe level (e.g. >1.0-1.5 G/L after the expected nadir, or PNN >0.5 G/L stable over 2-3 consecutive days).

o **Pegfilgrastim/Lipegfilgrastim (long-acting) :**

- Single fixed dose per cycle (e.g. Pegfilgrastim 6 mg SC).
- Administration: Usually 24 hours after the end of chemotherapy. Some on-body injector systems allow automated administration at the right time.
- **Do not administer within 14 days of the next chemotherapy cycle** (for pegfilgrastim, due to its long half-life).

- 11.5.2 Side-effects of G-CSF :

Generally well tolerated, but some side effects may occur

o **Joint and muscle pain (myalgia):** Most frequent side effect, especially with pegylated forms. Generally moderate and relieved by simple analgesics (paracetamol, NSAIDs if no contraindication). The use of antihistamines (e.g. loratadine) has been suggested to prevent/treat these pains [1, 2].

o Transient fever, headache.

o Injection site reactions (pain, redness).

o Elevation of LDH, PAL, uric acid (reversible).

o Splenomegaly (rare, especially with prolonged use).

o Splenic rupture (exceptional).

o Capillary leak syndrome (very rare).

o Significant leukocytosis (PNN >50-100 G/L): may require temporary interruption of G-CSF.

o Theoretical risk (not clearly demonstrated clinically for G-CSF used in oncology) of stimulating the growth of certain myeloid tumours (acute myeloid leukaemia - AML). Caution and discussion in cases of AML.

Table 11.2: Main side-effects of G-CSF and their management

(Source: Original creation based on RCP and literature [1, 2])

Side effect	Frequency	Recommended management	Comments
Osteoarticular pain/myalgia	Very frequent (30-50%)	- Analgesics (paracetamol, NSAIDs if no IC). - Antihistamines (loratadine) for prevention.	More marked with pegylated forms. Generally transient (48-72h).
Injection site reactions	Common (10-20%)	- Application of cold. - Rotation of injection sites.	Redness, local pain. Resolves in 1-2 days.
Transient fever	Occasional (5-10%)	- Monitoring. - Antipyretics if necessary.	Differentiate from febrile neutropenia (NF).
Headache	Occasional (5-15%)	- Paracetamol. - Hydration.	Linked to immune activation.
Marked leukocytosis (PNN >50 G/L)	Rare	- Temporary discontinuation of G-CSF. - Blood count monitoring.	Theoretical risk of thrombotic complications.
Splenomegaly	Rare (<1%)	- Ultrasound if symptoms (left hypochondrium pain). - Discontinue G-CSF if severe.	Monitor in case of prolonged use.

Splenic rupture	Exceptional	- Surgical emergency.	Warning signs: sudden abdominal pain, hypotension.
Capillary leak syndrome	Very rare	- Immediate discontinuation of G-CSF. - Intensive care management.	ffidema, hypotension, haemoconcentration.
Elevation of LDH/PAL	Common (asymptomatic)	- No specific treatment. - Biological monitoring.	Reversible on discontinuation.
Theoretical risk of AML	Contradictory data	- Avoid in case of proven AML. - Benefit/risk to be discussed in cases of predisposition.	No clear link in solid oncology. Caution in haemopathies.

11.6 Recommendations from learned societies (ASCO, ESMO, NCCN, EORTC)

The main international learned societies have issued recommendations for the use of G-CSF in oncology [1, 4, 5, 7]. Although there are slight variations, the general principles are consistent:

- **Primary prophylaxis:** Recommended if NF risk >20% (or 10-20% with patient risk factors). The objective of chemotherapy (curative) reinforces the indication.
- **Secondary prophylaxis:** Recommended after an episode of NF without primary prophylaxis, if maintenance of dose intensity is desired.
- **Therapeutic use:** Not routinely recommended. To be considered on a case-by-case basis for patients at very high risk of complications.
- **Choice of G-CSF**: Long-acting (pegylated) forms are often preferred for their convenience (a single injection per cycle), but short-acting forms remain a valid option. The choice may also depend on economic considerations and the availability of biosimilars.
- **Timing of administration:** It is vital to respect the timing of chemotherapy.
- These recommendations are regularly updated. It is important to refer to the most recent versions.

Table 11.3: Summary table of recommendations from learned societies (ASCO, ESMO, NCCN, EORTC) on the use of G-CSF

(Source: Summary of guidelines ASCO 2023, ESMO 2022, NCCN v3.2024, EORTC 2021 [1,4, 5, 7])

Aspect	ASCO (2023)	ESMO (2022)	NCCN (2024)	EORTC (2021)
Primary prophylaxis	**- Recommended** if NF risk >20%. **- Considered** if risk 10-20% + patient risk factors.	- Same as ASCO. - Emphasises assessment of **vital risk** (e.g. sepsis).	- Classifies protocols by risk level (High/Intermediate/Bas). - Specifies high-risk regimens by type of cancer.	- Emphasises **dose-dense protocols** (e.g. breast, lymphoma).
Secondary prophylaxis	**- Recommended** after an episode of NF if maintenance of dose-intensity is required.	**- Recommended** unless palliative chemotherapy with low benefit.	**- Recommended** after NF, with possible adjustment of chemotherapy protocol.	**- Recommended** especially for **curative** treatments.
Choice of G-CSF	**- Pegylates preferred** (commodity). - Biosimilars encouraged.	- No preference between pegylated/non-pegylated. - Cost to be considered.	- Pegfilgrastim **preferred** for primary prophylaxis.	- Short forms possible if closely monitored.
Timing of administration	- **24h post-chemotherapy** (not before 24h). s before 24h). - Avoid 14 days before the next cycle.	- Identical to ASCO. - Precise: **12-24h** for taxanes.	- **24-72h** for short forms. - **Strictly 24h** for pegylates.	- Insists on avoidance of **chemotherapy days**.
Therapeutic use	**- Not recommended** except in special cases (e.g. NF with sepsis).	**- Limited to** patients at very high risk of complications.	**- On a case-by-case basis** (e.g. severe comorbidities).	**- Not recommended** for routine use.
Special populations	**- Age >65 years**: risk threshold reduced to 10% if comorbidities.	**- Fragile patients**: prophylaxis even if intermediate risk.	**- Haematological cancers**: specific rules (e.g. AML).	**- Paediatrics**: dosage adjustments.

Conclusion

Granulocyte growth factors (G-CSF) are essential pharmacological tools in the prevention of chemotherapy-induced febrile neutropenia. Their judicious use in primary prophylaxis, based on a rigorous assessment of the risk associated with the treatment and the patient, makes it possible to significantly reduce the incidence of NF, maintain the dose-intensity of chemotherapy (especially in curative situations), and improve patient safety. Secondary prophylaxis is also a well-established indication. However, their role in therapeutic situations (established NF) remains limited to selected cases. The availability of long-acting G-CSF and biosimilars has changed practices and economic considerations. A good knowledge of the indications, administration methods and potential side-effects of G-CSFs is essential for all clinicians involved in oncology.

References

1. Smith TJ, Bohlke K, Lyman GH, et al. Recommendations for the Use of WBC Growth Factors: American Society of Clinical Oncology Clinical Practice Guideline Update. J Clin Oncol. 2015;33(28):3199-3212.
2. Aapro MS, Cameron DA, Pettengell R, et al. EORTC guidelines for the use of granulocyte-colony stimulating factor to reduce the incidence of chemotherapy-induced febrile neutropenia in adult patients with SCLC, GCT and NHL. Eur J Cancer. 2006;42(15):2433-2453.
3. Blackwell K, Semiglazov V, Krasnozhon D, et al. Comparison of Lipegfilgrastim Versus Pegfilgrastim in Patients With Breast Cancer Receiving Myelosuppressive Chemotherapy: Results of the Phase III Double-Blind, Randomized, Active-Control NEXES Trial. Oncologist. 2015;20(11):1285-1292.
4. Klastersky J, de Naurois J, Rolston K, et al. Management of febrile neutropaenia: ESMO Clinical Practice Guidelines. Ann Oncol. 2016;27(suppl 5):v111-v118.
5. National Comprehensive Cancer Network (NCCN). Clinical Practice Guidelines in Oncology: Hematopoietic Growth Factors. Version 1.2025.
6. Garcia-Carbonero R, Mayordomo JI, Tornamira MV, et al. Granulocyte colony-stimulating factor in the treatment of high-risk febrile neutropenia: a multicenter randomized trial. J Natl Cancer Inst. 2001;93(1):31-38.
7. Aapro MS, Bohlius J, Cameron DA, et al. 2010 update of EORTC guidelines for the use of granulocyte-colony stimulating factor to reduce the incidence of chemotherapy-induced febrile neutropenia in adult patients with lymphoproliferative disorders and solid tumours. Eur J Cancer. 2011;47(1):8-32.

Chapter 12: Anti-infective prophylaxis in patients at risk of cancer

Introduction

In addition to the use of granulocyte growth factors (G-CSF) to reduce the duration and depth of neutropenia, targeted anti-infective prophylaxis strategies may be considered for certain cancer patients at high risk of specific infections. These prophylaxes aim to prevent bacterial, fungal, viral or *Pneumocystis jirovecii* infections during periods of maximum immune vulnerability [1, 2]. However, their use must be judicious and based on a rigorous assessment of the benefit/risk ratio, taking into account the patient's individual risk, the type of anti-cancer treatment, and the potential for side-effects or the emergence of resistance [3]. This chapter details the indications, molecules, benefits and risks of the main anti-infective prophylaxes, as well as the importance of vaccinations.

12.1 Antibacterial prophylaxis

The aim of antibacterial prophylaxis is to reduce the incidence of bacterial infections and febrile neutropenia (NF) in high-risk patients. Fluoroquinolones are the most widely studied agents in this indication.

- 12.1.1 Indications and target populations :

Routine antibacterial prophylaxis is NOT recommended for all patients receiving myelotoxic chemotherapy due to the risk of side effects and selection of resistance [1, 3, 4]. It should be considered primarily in patients at high risk of NF and/or serious infectious complications, including:

- Patients with haematological malignancies receiving intensive induction chemotherapy (e.g. acute myeloid leukaemia - AML) or awaiting bone marrow recovery after haematopoietic stem cell (HSC) transplantation, especially if profound (PNN <0.1 G/L) and prolonged (>7-10 days) neutropenia is expected.
- Patients with solid tumours receiving chemotherapy regimens at very high risk of NF and severe mucositis, or with major additional risk factors (case-by-case decision).
- It is generally not routinely recommended for low-risk patients or those receiving regimens with an intermediate risk of NF, except in very specific situations.

- 12.1.2 Choice of Molecules and Modalities :

- Fluoroquinolones (FQ) :
  - Levofloxacin (500 mg x 1/day PO) or Ciprofloxacin (500 mg x 2/day PO) are the most widely used.
  - They have good activity against many Gram-negative bacilli (GNB), but variable activity against Gram-positive cocci (GPC) and anaerobes.

■ Onset: Generally at the start of the expected period of neutropenia (or as early as Day 1 of chemotherapy for certain very high-risk protocols).

■ Duration: Maintained for the duration of severe neutropenia (PNN <0.5 G/L) or until haematological recovery.

- 12.1.3 Benefits and Risks :

o Demonstrated benefits in high-risk populations:

■ Reduced incidence of febrile episodes.

■ Reduced incidence of bacteremia (especially BGN).

■ Possible reduction in infection-related mortality in some studies and meta-analyses, but this point is more debated [1, 4].

o Risks and disadvantages :

■ Selection of bacterial resistance: This is the major concern. The widespread use of FQs may encourage the emergence of resistant strains (FQ-resistant BGN, *Clostridioides difficile*). The impact on local and individual bacterial ecology must be taken into account.

■ Side effects of FQs: Digestive disorders, tendinopathy (tendon rupture), QT prolongation, photosensitivity, neuropsychiatric effects.

■ Potential masking of early infection (delayed fever).

■ Cost.

o The decision to institute FQ prophylaxis must therefore be carefully weighed and reserved for situations where the expected benefit clearly outweighs the risks, taking into account the local epidemiology of resistance.

12.2 Antifungal prophylaxis

The aim is to prevent invasive fungal infections (IFIs), particularly candidiasis and aspergillosis, in very high-risk patients.

12.2.1 Indications and target populations :

Routine antifungal prophylaxis is only justified in very selected groups of patients at very high risk of IFI [1, 3, 5, 6]:

o Patients with high-risk acute myeloid leukaemia (AML) or myelodysplastic syndrome (MDS) receiving intensive induction or consolidation chemotherapy, and in whom profound and prolonged neutropenia (>10-14 days) is expected.

o HSC allograft recipients during the post-graft neutropenia phase and/or in cases of acute or extensive chronic graft-versus-host disease (GVHD) treated with immunosuppressants.

o It is not generally recommended routinely for patients with solid tumours or those receiving less intensive chemotherapy, even if neutropenia is expected.

- 12.2.2 Choice of Molecules and Modalities :

The choice of prophylactic agent depends on the type of fungus you wish to cover (yeasts alone, or yeasts and moulds).

o Anti-Candida prophylaxis (mainly) :

■ Fluconazole (400 mg x 1/day PO or IV): Effective in preventing invasive candidiasis in high-risk patients (e.g. allograft recipients). Has no activity on moulds (*Aspergillus spp*., Mucorales).

o Anti-Candida AND anti-Aspergillus (mould) prophylaxis :

■ Posaconazole (gastro-resistant tablets 300 mg x 1/day PO, or oral suspension, or IV form): Broad-spectrum azole, effective as prophylaxis in induction AML/MDS patients and allograft recipients with GVH [5, 6].

■ Voriconazole (200 mg x 2/day PO or IV): Alternative to posaconazole, but more drug interactions and toxicity (hepatic, visual).

■ Itraconazole (oral solution): Efficacy limited by erratic bioavailability and poor digestive tolerance. Less widely used.

■ Micafungin (echinocandin IV): May be an option for certain patients intolerant of azoles or at high risk of azole-resistant candidiasis, but its anti-Aspergillus spectrum is less robust than that of new-generation azoles.

o Initiation: Usually with chemotherapy or at the onset of neutropenia.

o Duration: Maintained throughout the high-risk period (profound and prolonged neutropenia, major immunosuppression).

- 12.2.3 Benefits and Risks :

o Benefit: Reduction in the incidence of proven IFI and IFI-related mortality in very high-risk populations.

o Risks:

■ Toxicity of antifungal agents (hepatotoxicity of azoles, nephrotoxicity of amphotericin B if used).

■ Numerous drug interactions with azoles (via cytochrome P450).

■ Selection of resistant fungal strains (e.g. fluconazole-resistant *Candida glabrata* or *krusei*, azole-resistant *Aspergillus*).

■ Cost

Table 12.1: Antifungal prophylactic options (summary)

Agent	Spectrum	Dosage	Advantages	Limitations
Fluconazole	Candida (non-albicans resistant)	400 mg/day PO/IV	Good tolerance, moderate cost	Inactive on Aspergillus, resistance possible
Posaconazole	Candida + Aspergillus	300 mg/day PO/IV	Broad spectrum, reduces mortality (AML)	Interactions, high cost
Voriconazole	Candida + Aspergillus Aspergillus	200 mg x 2/d PO/IV	Alternative to posaconazole	Toxicity (hepatic, neurological)

Micafungin	Candida (partial aspergillosis)	50 mg/d IV	No interactions CYP450	Limited spectrum, IV administration

Decision algorithm for antifungal prophylaxis in neutropenic patients neutropenic patient

(Source: Adapted from ECIL-8, ESCMID 2023, IDSA 2024 [1, 3, 6, 7])

Steps in the algorithm

1. **IFI risk assessment** :

○ **Very high risk** (systematic prophylaxis recommended):

■ Induction/consolidation AML/MDS (neutropenia >10-14 days).

■ HSC allograft (neutropenia phase or treated GVH).

○ **Intermediate risk** (prophylaxis to be discussed):

■ HSC autograft with risk factors (e.g. severe mucositis).

■ Intensive chemotherapy for lymphoma.

○ **Low risk** (prophylaxis not recommended):

■ Short neutropenia (<7 days) or solid tumours.

2. **Choice of antifungal agent** :

○ **Anti-Candida alone** (if low risk of aspergillosis) :

■ Fluconazole 400 mg/d (PO/IV).

○ **Anti-Candida + Anti-Aspergillus** (if high risk of mould) :

■ **Posaconazole** (300 mg/d PO/IV): 1st line (grade A).

■ **Voriconazole** (200 mg x 2/d PO/IV): Alternative.

■ **Micafungin** (50 mg/d IV): If intolerant to azoles.

3. **Practical details** :

○ **Start**: Day 1 of chemotherapy or onset of neutropenia.

○ **Duration**: Until recovery of PNN (>0.5 G/L) or end of immunosuppression.

○ **Monitoring**:

■ Liver function tests (azoles).

■ Drug interactions (check for CYP3A4 substrates).

12.3 Antiviral prophylaxis (HSV, VZV)

The aim is to prevent reactivation of the Herpes Simplex virus (HSV) and Varicella-Zoster virus (VZV).

- 12.3.1 Indications and target populations :

○ HSV-positive patients receiving induction chemotherapy for acute leukaemiaê or HSC transplantation (autograft or allograft), especially if severe mucositis is expected [1, 3, 7].

○ VZV-positive patients (history of chickenpox or herpes zoster) at high risk of reactivation:

■ HSC allograft recipients.

■ Treatment with certain highly immunosuppressive agents (e.g. alemtuzumab, bortezomib, BTK inhibitors, fludarabine).

■ Certain patients with lymphoma or multiple myeloma.

• 12.3.2 Choice of molecules and modalities :

○ Aciclovir (200-400 mg x 2-3/day PO or 250 mg/m^{2}x 2-3/day IV).

◦ Valaciclovir (500 mg x 1-2/day PO), a pro-drug of aciclovir with better bioavailability.

◦ Start: At the beginning of the period of maximum immunosuppression.

◦ Duration: As long as immunosuppression persists (e.g. several months after transplantation, or for the duration of treatment at risk).

- **12.3.3 Benefits and Risks :**

◦ Benefits: Very effective in preventing HSV and VZV reactivations and their complications.

◦ Risks: Generally well tolerated. Possible renal toxicity with high-dose IV aciclovir (crystalluria), especially if dehydrated or with pre-existing renal impairment. Rare but possible emergence of aciclovir resistance in highly immunocompromised patients on long-term treatment.

12.4 Anti-Pneumocystis jirovecii (PJP) prophylaxis

The aim is to prevent pulmonary pneumocystis (PCP), a potentially fatal opportunistic infection in immunocompromised patients.

- **12.4.1 Indications and target populations :**

Anti-PJP prophylaxis is recommended in patients at significant risk, including [1, 3, 8]:

◦ Patients receiving prolonged high-dose corticosteroid therapy (e.g. >20 mg/day prednisone equivalent for >4 weeks).

◦ Patients with acute lymphoblastic leukaemia (ALL).

◦ HSC allograft recipients (at least for the first 6 months and for as long as immunosuppression persists).

◦ Patients treated with certain immunosuppressive agents (e.g. fludarabine, alemtuzumab, temozolomide with concomitant radiotherapy for glioblastoma).

◦ Certain patients with lymphomas or other haematological malignancies undergoing specific treatments.

- **12.4.2 Choice of Molecules and Modalities :**

◦ Cotrimoxazole (Trimethoprim-Sulfamethoxazole, TMP-SMX): Treatment of choice.

▪ Regimens: One strong tablet (160mg TMP/800mg SMX) 3 times/week (e.g. Monday-Wednesday-Friday) OR one single tablet (80mg TMP/400mg SMX) per day.

◦ Alternatives in cases of intolerance or contraindication to cotrimoxazole:

▪ Dapsone (100mg/day PO or 50mg x2/day PO). Requires verification of absence of G6PD deficiency.

▪ Atovaquone (1500 mg/day PO oral suspension).

▪ Pentamidine aerosol (300 mg every 4 weeks). Less effective for extrapulmonary prophylaxis, may induce bronchospasm.

- Duration: As long as the immunosuppression risk factor persists.

- 12.4.3 Benefits and Risks :

- Benefit: Very effective in preventing PCP.
- Risks:

■ Cotrimoxazole: Cutaneous rash (sometimes severe), digestive disorders, cytopenias (increased myelosuppression), hyperkalaemia, renal failure.

■ Dapsone: Haemolysis (especially if G6PD deficiency), methaemoglobinaemia, agranulocytosis (rare).

■ Atovaquone: Digestive disorders, rash.

■ Pentamidine aerosol: Cough, bronchospasm.

12.5 Vaccinations in cancer patients

Vaccination is an important means of preventing certain infections in cancer patients, whose immunity may be compromised by the disease or its treatment.

- **12.5.1 General principles :**

- Ideally, vaccinations should be updated before the start of immunosuppressive cancer treatment, when the immune response is still optimal.
- Inactivated (killed) vaccines: Generally safe in immunocompromised patients, although their efficacy may be reduced. Examples: influenza, pneumococcus, COVID-19, hepatitis B, dTap (diphtheria-tetanus-pertussis).
- Live attenuated vaccines: Generally contraindicated during periods of significant immunosuppression (chemotherapy, high-dose corticosteroid therapy, etc.) due to the risk of disseminated infection by the vaccine strain. Examples: MMR (measles-mumps-rubella), varicella-zoster (live VZV vaccine), yellow fever, BCG. The recombinant inactivated shingles vaccine (Shingrix®) is an option for patients aged over 50, including immunocompromised patients.

- **12.5.2 Specific recommendations :**

- Influenza vaccine: Recommended annually for all cancer patients and their close contacts. Can be administered during chemotherapy (ideally between courses).
- Pneumococcal vaccines: Recommended (PCV13 or PCV15/20 conjugate vaccine followed by PPSV23 polysaccharide vaccine) for patients at risk, particularly before or after splenectomy, or in the event of immunosuppression.
- Anti-COVID-19 vaccine: Strongly recommended (full schedule and boosters) in accordance with national recommendations.

o Other vaccines: Depending on previous vaccination status, specific risks and current recommendations (e.g. *Haemophilus influenzae* type b, meningococcus in asplenics).

Table 12.2: Recommended vaccinations for adult cancer patients

(Source: Adapted from IDSA 2023, CDC 2024, HCSP 2023 recommendations)

Vaccine	Type	Specific recommendations	Ideal timing	Contra-indications/Precautions
Influenza (inactivated)	Inactivated	**Annually** for all patients and their families.	Between cycles of chemotherapy.	Avoid during severe neutropenia (<0.5 G/L).
Pneumococcus	Conjugate (PCV13/15/20)	**PCV13/15/20** followed by **PPSV23** (at 8 weeks) for immunocompromised patients.	Before treatment if possible.	No restriction on immunosuppression.
COVID-19	mRNA/inactivated	**Complete regimen + boosters** according to national guidelines.	At any time (priority between cycles).	None (except severe allergy to components).
dTap (diphtheria-tetanus-pertussis)	Inactivated	**Booster every 10 years** (dT). Whooping cough if in contact with infants.	Before treatment.	None.
Hepatitis B	Inactivated	If seronegative (anti-HBs <10 UI/L) and risk of exposure. Accelerated regimen possible (0-1-2-6 months).	Before immunosuppression.	Reduced efficacy under immunosuppressants.
Shingles (Shingrix®)	Recombinant subunit	**Recommended** for people over 50 (including immunocompromised patients). 2 doses at 2-6 months.	During stable periods.	Avoid during intensive chemotherapy.
MMR (measles-mumps-rubella)	Live attenuated	**Contraindicated** during immunosuppression. À administer **4 weeks before** treatment if possible.	Only before immunosuppression.	Neutropenia, immunosuppression severe.
Varicella (VZV) during	Live attenuated	**Contraindicated** immunosuppression. For non-immune patients, check IgG before treatment.	Before treatment.	Same as MMR.
Yellow fever	Live attenuated essential	**Avoid** except for travel to endemic areas (discussed on a case-by-case basis).	Only if essential.	Risk of disseminated vaccine disease.

- 12.5.3 Vaccine response :

The immune response to vaccines may be reduced in patients undergoing chemotherapy or other immunosuppressive treatments. The optimal time for vaccination (before, during, after treatment) should be discussed with the oncologist. Post-vaccination serological testing is not generally performed routinely, except in special situations.

Conclusion

Targeted anti-infective prophylaxis strategies, including the use of antibiotics, antifungals, antivirals and anti-PJP prophylaxis, play an important role in reducing infectious morbidity and mortality in selected subgroups of high-risk cancer patients during periods of neutropenia or profound immunosuppression. However, these prophylaxes are not without risks (side-effects, emergence of resistance) and their indications must be rigorously assessed on a case-by-case basis, based on the recommendations of learned societies and the patient's individual risk profile. At the same time, a proactive vaccination policy aimed at protecting patients against vaccine-preventable infections is an essential component of oncology support care. The decision to introduce prophylaxis should always be based on an individualised risk/benefit balance.

References

1. Freifeld AG, Bow EJ, Sepkowitz KA, et al. Clinical practice guideline for the use of antimicrobial agents in neutropenic patients with cancer: 2010 update by the Infectious Diseases Society of America. Clin Infect Dis. 2011;52(4):e56-e93.

2. Baden LR, Swaminathan S, Angarone M, et al. Prevention and Treatment of Cancer-Related Infections, Version 2.2016, NCCN Clinical Practice Guidelines in Oncology. J Natl Compr Canc Netw. 2016;14(7):882-913.

3. Klastersky J, de Naurois J, Rolston K, et al. Management of febrile neutropaenia: ESMO Clinical Practice Guidelines. Ann Oncol. 2016;27(suppl 5):v111-v118.

4. Gafter-Gvili A, Fraser A, Paul M, Leibovici L. Antibiotic prophylaxis for bacterial infections in afebrile neutropenic patients following chemotherapy. Cochrane Database Syst Rev. 2012;(1):CD004386.

5. Maertens JA, Girmenia C, Bruggemann RJ, et al. European Conference on Infections in Leukaemia (ECIL-6) guidelines for the treatment of invasive candidiasis, aspergillosis and mucormycosis in leukemia and hematopoietic stem cell transplant patients. Haematologica. 2018;103(3):e81-e83.

6. Cornely OA, Maertens J, Winston DJ, et al. Posaconazole vs. fluconazole or itraconazole for prophylaxis of invasive fungal infections in patients with neutropenia from myelodysplastic syndromes or acute myeloid leukemia. N Engl J Med. 2007;356(4):348-359.

7. Tomblyn M, Chiller T, Einsele H, et al. Guidelines for preventing infectious complications among hematopoietic cell transplantation recipients: a global perspective. Biol Blood Marrow Transplant. 2009;15(10):1143-1238.

8. Cooley L, Dendle C, Wolf J, et al. Consensus guidelines for diagnosis, prophylaxis and management of Pneumocystis jirovecii pneumonia in patients with haematological and solid malignancies, 2014. Intern Med J. 2014;44(12b):1350-1363.

Part 5

Special Situations and Perspectives Chapter 13: Febrile Neutropenia in the Elderly Introduction

The ageing of the population is accompanied by an increase in the incidence of cancer in the elderly (generally defined as those aged 65-70 and over). Although chronological age alone is not a contraindication to cancer treatment, elderly patients represent a heterogeneous population with physiological specificities, frequent comorbidities, polymedication and potential frailty that may influence treatment tolerance and the management of complications, particularly febrile neutropenia (NF) [1, 2]. This chapter focuses on the particularities of the clinical presentation of NF in elderly patients, the impact of comorbidities and polymedication, the necessary adaptations in risk stratification and therapeutic strategies, and the importance of managing frailty.

13.1 Specificities of the Clinical Presentation of Febrile Neutropenia in the Elderly Patient

The clinical presentation of NF and underlying infections may be atypical or attenuated in the elderly patient, sometimes making diagnosis more difficult [3, 4].

- **Reduced or absent fever:**
  - Elderly patients may have a less marked or even absent febrile response, even in the presence of severe infection. Hypothermia can sometimes be a sign of severe infection.
  - The classic definition of fever (>38.3°C or >38°C for 1 hour) should be interpreted with caution. A rise in temperature >1°C above the patient's basal temperature, even if <38°C, should raise the alarm.
- **Non-specific or misleading symptoms:**
  - Fatigue, anorexia, confusion, agitation, falls, or a deterioration in general condition may be the only signs of an incipient infection, and may be mistakenly attributed to ageing or cancerous disease.
  - Pain may be less well expressed or localised.
  - The classic signs of local inflammation (redness, heat, swelling) may be less obvious.
- **Presentation of Specific Organs :**
  - **Pulmonary infection:** less productive cough, dyspnoea sometimes interpreted as an exacerbation of COPD or heart failure. Chest X-ray may be less informative initially.
  - **Urinary tract infection:** Confusion, incontinence, or simple alteration of general condition may be the only signs, without the classic mictional

burning.
○ **Skin infection:** Less obvious local inflammatory signs.
• **Consequences:** These atypical presentations can lead to delays in diagnosis and treatment, with a potentially negative impact on prognosis. Increased vigilance and a low threshold of suspicion are therefore necessary.

Table 13.1: Signs of infection in young versus elderly neutropenic patients

Parameter	Young patient (<65 years)	Elderly patient (>65 years)	Clinical implications
Febrile response	Well marked fever >38.3°C	Fever absent/attenuated (± hypothermia)	Diagnostic threshold lowered to +1°C above basal level
General symptoms	Fatigue/clear localisation of symptoms	Isolated confusion/falls/anorexia	Systematic search for an infectious source in the event of any change in general condition
Pulmonary signs	Productive cough, chest pain	Isolated dyspnoea (mimicking COPD/cardiac decompensation)	Early chest CT scan if in doubt
Urinary signs	Urinary urgency, pollakiuria	Incontinence/aggravation of cognitive impairment	Systematic ECBU even without urinary symptoms
Biological markers	Elevated CRP, hyperleukocytosis (if not neutropenic)	Attenuated infiammatone response	**Clombination** with procalcitonin and clinical course

13.2 Impact of Comorbidities and Polymedication

Elderly patients frequently present with multiple comorbidities and polymedication, which complicates the management of NF [1, 2, 5].

• **Common comorbidities :**
○ Cardiovascular disease (heart failure, coronary artery disease, hypertension).
○ Chronic lung disease (COPD).
○ Chronic renal failure.
○ Diabetes.
○ Cognitive disorders, dementia.
○ malnutrition.
• **Impact of co-morbidities:** ○ Increase the risk of serious complications of NF and infections (e.g. cardiac decompensation, acute respiratory failure, additional ARF).
○ May limit therapeutic options (e.g. choice of antibiotics in renal failure, caution with vascular filling in heart failure).
○ May mask or mimic the symptoms of an infection.
• **Polymedication :**
○ **Increased risk of drug interactions:** between antibiotics, support

treatments and the patient's usual medication.

○ **Increased risk of drug side-effects:** due to pharmacokinetic and pharmacodynamic changes associated with age and co-morbidities.

○ Need for careful, regular review of prescriptions to optimise treatments and avoid harmful interactions. Collaboration with the clinical pharmacist is often useful.

13.3 Adapting risk and treatment stratification

Although the general principles of risk stratification and treatment of NF apply, adaptations are necessary in the elderly patient [1, 3, 5, 6].

- 13.3.1 Risk stratification :

○ Age > 65-70 is often considered an independent risk factor for complications in scores such as the MASCC, but it should be interpreted in the light of the patient's overall physiological state (frailty, comorbidities) rather than chronological age alone.

○ An in-depth geriatric assessment (EGA) can help to better assess the patient's individual risk and functional reserves.

○ Elderly patients, even with an initially reassuring MASCC score, may deteriorate more rapidly. Closer monitoring is often warranted.

○ The decision to manage patients on an outpatient basis must be particularly cautious, ensuring excellent social support and rapid access to care.

- 13.3.2 Choice and adaptation of antibiotic therapy :

○ The general recommendations on the choice of antibiotics (anti-pseudomonas coverage for high-risk patients) remain valid.

○ **Dosage must be adjusted according to renal function:** creatinine clearance is often reduced in elderly patients, even with normal creatinine levels (reduced muscle mass). The use of formulas such as Cockcroft-Gault or MDRD/CKD-EPI is essential for estimating renal function and adjusting doses of renally eliminated antibiotics (beta-lactams, aminoglycosides, vancomycin, etc.) to avoid toxic accumulation.

○ **Caution with certain antibiotics:**

■ Aminosides: Increased risk of nephrotoxicity and ototoxicity. Use on for short periods, with monitoring of levels if possible.

■ Fluoroquinolones: Increased risk of tendinopathy, neuropsychiatric disorders and QT prolongation.

■ Vancomycin: Risk of nephrotoxicity. Monitor serum levels.

○ Prefer the simplest and best tolerated regimens if possible.

. 13.3.3 Use of G-CSF :

○ Primary prophylaxis with G-CSF is often more widely indicated in elderly patients receiving chemotherapy regimens with an intermediate risk of NF

(10-20%), due to their increased vulnerability [1, 6].

o The therapeutic use of G-CSF in elderly patients with established NF may be considered more liberally, especially if poor prognostic factors are present.

- 13.3.4 Supportive care :

o Hydration: Careful monitoring of hydration status, as the risk of dehydration is increased. Cautious vascular filling if cardiac insufficiency.

o Nutrition: Early detection and management of malnutrition.

o Prevention of decubitus complications in the event of prolonged hospitalisation.

13.4 Frailty management and the geriatric oncology approach

Frailty is a common geriatric syndrome, characterised by reduced physiological reserves and increased vulnerability to stress, which is distinct from chronological age and comorbidities [2, 5].

- **13.4.1 Identifying frailty:**

o Use of validated frailty scales (e.g. Fried score, Clinical Frailty Scale, G8 screening tool).

o An in-depth geriatric assessment (IGA) by a geriatrician or a mobile geriatric team can identify areas of frailty (functional, cognitive, nutritional, social, psychological) and propose a personalised care plan.

- **13.4.2 Implications of frailty for NF management:**

o Fragile patients are at increased risk of NF complications, functional decline, loss of autonomy and mortality.

o They are less tolerant of aggressive treatments and their side effects.

o The therapeutic decision must take into account the assessment of frailty and the patient's care objectives (quality of life, maintenance of autonomy).

- **13.4.3 Geriatric Oncology Approach (GOA) :**

o Collaboration between oncologists and geriatricians is essential to optimise the care of elderly cancer patients, including the management of la NF.

o AGO aims to:

▪ Adapt cancer treatments and toxicity management based on geriatric assessment.

▪ Prevent functional and cognitive decline.

▪ Optimise nutrition and social support.

▪ Incorporate patient preferences into care decisions.

Conclusion

The management of febrile neutropenia in elderly patients requires an individualised approach that takes account of the specific features of this population. Atypical clinical presentations, the impact of co-morbidities and multi-medication, and the frequent presence of a frailty syndrome make diagnosis and treatment more complex. Adaptation of risk stratification strategies, judicious choice of antibiotics with dosage adjustment according to renal function, and wider use of G-CSF prophylaxis are key elements. A multidisciplinary approach, integrating geriatric expertise within a geriatric oncology approach, is fundamental to optimising management, preserving autonomy and quality of life, and improving the prognosis of these vulnerable patients.

References

1. Aapro MS, Bohlius J, Cameron DA, et al. 2010 update of EORTC guidelines for the use of granulocyte-colony stimulating factor to reduce the incidence of chemotherapy-induced febrile neutropenia in adult patients with lymphoproliferative disorders and solid tumours. Eur J Cancer. 2011;47(1):8-32.
2. Wildiers H, Heeren P, Puts M, et al. International Society of Geriatric Oncology consensus on geriatric assessment in older patients with cancer. J Clin Oncol. 2014;32(24):2595-2603.
3. Klastersky J. Management of fever in neutropenic patients with special emphasis on the elderly. Clin Infect Dis. 2004;39 Suppl 1:S52-S57.
4. High KP, Bradley SF, Gravenstein S, et al. Clinical practice guideline for the evaluation of fever and infection in older adult residents of long-term care facilities: 2008 update by the Infectious Diseases Society of America. Clin Infect Dis. 2009;48(2):149-171.
5. Lyman GH, Dale DC, Culakova E, et al. The impact of chemotherapy dose intensity on cancer patient outcomes: a systematic review. J Clin Oncol. 2005;23(36_suppl):8500-8500.
6. Taplitz RA, Kennedy EB, Bow EJ, et al. Outpatient Management of Febrile Neutropenia in Adults Treated for Malignancy: American Society of Clinical Oncology and Infectious Diseases Society of America Clinical Practice Guideline Update. J Clin Oncol. 2018;36(14):1443-1453.

Chapter 14: Febrile Neutropenia in Haematologic Malignancies

Introduction

Patients with haematological malignancies, such as acute leukaemias, aggressive lymphomas, or those receiving haematopoietic stem cell (HSC) transplantation, are a particularly vulnerable population to febrile neutropenia (NF) and its infectious complications [1]. Because of the nature of their disease and the intensity of the cytotoxic or immunosuppressive treatments they receive, these patients often develop **deeper and more prolonged neutropenia** than those seen in solid tumours [2]. This context of severe and long-lasting immunodepression exposes them to a **particular risk of infection**, with a wider spectrum of pathogens and often more serious infections. This chapter focuses on the **specific features of NF in haematological malignancies**, addressing the characteristics of neutropenia, the profile of infections, and the particularities of therapeutic and prophylactic management.

14.1 Characteristics of neutropenia in haematological malignancies

- 14.1.1 Profound and prolonged neutropenia :

○ **Acute myeloid leukaemia (AML) and lymphoblastic leukaemia (ALL):** Induction and consolidation chemotherapy for AML almost systematically induces bone marrow aplasia with profound (PNN < 0.1 G/L) and prolonged (often > 14-21 days) neutropenia [3, 4]. Recovery of bone marrow may be slow.

○ **Haematopoietic Stem Cell (HSC) transplant :**

■ **HSC autograft:** Myeloablative conditioning leads to profound neutropenia, generally lasting 7 to 14 days until recovery from aplasia.

■ **HSC allograft**: Post-conditioning neutropenia is also profound and may be prolonged, especially in cases of delayed engraftment. In addition, immunosuppression induced to prevent or treat graft-versus-host disease (GVHD) contributes to a global and long-lasting immune deficiency [5].

○ **Aggressive lymphomas and multiple myeloma:** Some intensive chemotherapy regimens may also induce severe and prolonged neutropenia.

• **14.1.2 Qualitative alteration of PNN :**

In addition to the simple quantitative reduction, the haematological disease itself (e.g. myelodysplasia, leukaemia) or certain treatments may alter the function of residual NPCs (lack of phagocytosis, chemotaxis).

• **14.1.3 Impairment of Other Lineages and Cellular/Humoral Immunity :**

Patients with haematological malignancies often present a more global immunodepression, with lymphopenia (T, B, NK), impaired humoral immunity (hypogammaglobulinaemia, particularly in myeloma or CLL), and macrophage dysfunction, increasing the risk of infection.

14.2 Particular infectious risk: spectrum of pathogens

The depth and duration of neutropenia, together with overall immunosuppression, expose these patients to a wider spectrum of infections and to more severe infections [1, 2, 6].

- **14.2.1 Bacterial infections :**

○ **Gram-negative bacilli (GNB):** Still a major cause of serious infections and bacteraemia (digestive translocation favoured by severe mucositis). *Pseudomonas aeruginosa* and enterobacteria (including ESBL and carbapenemase producers) are particularly dreaded.

○ **Gram-positive cocci (PGC):** High incidence, particularly infections associated with central catheters (staphylococci, enterococci). Streptococci of the *viridans* group (oropharyngeal translocation during mucositis, risk of septic shock and ARDS).

○ Anaerobic infections (if mucositis, neutropenic enterocolitis).

- **14.2.2 Invasive Fungal Infections (IFI) :**

○ **Very high risk**, especially if profound neutropenia >10-14 days, GVH, corticosteroid therapy.

○ **Invasive candidiasis (candidaemia, disseminated hepatosplenic candidiasis):** *Candida albicans* and non-albicans species (e.g. *C. glabrata*, *C. krusei*, *C. parapsilosis*).

○ **Invasive pulmonary aspergillosis (IPA):** Mainly mould IFI. Can also be sinus or disseminated.

○ **Other moulds (rarer but often with a poor prognosis):** Mucorales (mucormycosis), Fusarium, Scedosporium.

- **14.2.3 Viral infections :**

○ **Reactivation of Herpesviridae:** HSV (herpetic mucositis), VZV (extensive/disseminated shingles), **CMV** (pneumopathy, colitis, hepatitis, especially after allogeneic transplantation or with alemtuzumab/fludarabine), EBV (lymphoproliferative syndromes).

○ **Respiratory viruses:** influenza, RSV, metapneumovirus, adenovirus (can cause severe and prolonged infections, particularly pneumonia).

○ More rarely: parvovirus B19 (erythroblastopenia), polyomavirus BK (haemorrhagic cystitis after transplantation).

- 14.2.4 Rare opportunistic infections / Polymicrobial infections :

Possible in cases of very profound and prolonged immunosuppression.

14.3 Specific features of diagnostic and therapeutic management

The management of NF in this context requires increased vigilance and often more aggressive strategies [1, 2, 3, 6, 7].

- **14.3.1 Initial assessment and risk stratification :**

o Most of these patients are immediately considered to be **at high risk of** complications due to the expected depth and duration of neutropenia, and co-morbidities associated with their haemopathy.

o The MASCC score is often <21 and less discriminating in this population. Other factors (type of haemopathy, phase of treatment, intensity of immunosuppression) are taken into account.

o Systematic hospitalisation.

- **14.3.2 Initial Empirical Antibiotic Therapy :**

o **Always intravenous and broad spectrum, with robust antipseudomonas activity.**

o Often, **dual therapy** (anti-pseudomonas beta-lactam + aminoglycoside) is preferred as first-line treatment, at least for the first 48-72 hours, because of the potential severity of BGN infections.

o **Carbapenems** may be used more frequently as a first-line treatment if there is a high risk of ESBL-producing BGN (local epidemiology, known colonisation).

o The use of **glycopeptides as first-line treatment** is debated, but is often more widespread, particularly in cases of severe mucositis, suspected catheter infection, or haemodynamic instability, due to the risk of infections with CGP (viridans streptococci, staphylococci).

- **14.3.3 Reassessment and adjustment of treatment :**

o If fever persists (>4-7 days) despite broad-spectrum antibiotic therapy:

■ Intensive search for an outbreak (systematic thoracic CT scan, other imaging if necessary).

■ **Early addition of a broad-spectrum empirical antifungal treatment** (covering *Aspergillus* and *Candida*, eg:
caspofungin, L-AMB, voriconazole - see Chapter 8) is common and recommended practice [6, 7].

■ Consider viral infections (CMV, respiratory viruses).

o De-escalation is possible but must be cautious, taking into account the persistence of profound neutropenia.

. **14.3.4 Use of G-CSF :**

o Primary and secondary prophylaxis: Widely used and recommended with intensive chemotherapy regimens for AML/ALL or aggressive lymphomas, and after HSC autotransplantation.

o Therapeutic use in established NF: More often considered in this high-risk population, especially if severe sepsis, proven fungal infection, or very prolonged expected neutropenia, although evidence of benefit on mortality remains limited [1, 5].

- **14.3.5 Diagnosis and management of IFI :**

o Active monitoring of fungal markers (Galactomannan, Beta-D-Glucan) in high-risk patients.

o Low threshold for chest CT.

o BAL and biopsies more often required.

o Prolonged curative antifungal treatment if IFI proven/probable.

- **14.3.6 Management of viral infections :**

o Monitoring of CMV viral load in allograft patients and other patients at risk. Pre-emptive treatment if significant reactivation occurs.

o Rapid diagnosis and treatment of HSV/VZV and respiratory virus infections.

14.4 Specific features of anti-infective prophylaxis

Because of the major risk of infection, anti-infective prophylaxis is more widely used and often combined in patients with haematological malignancies in the aplastic phase [1, 2, 3, 6, 7].

- **Antibacterial prophylaxis :**

o **Fluoroquinolones (levofloxacin):** Recommended in patients at high risk of profound and prolonged neutropenia (e.g. AML induction, HSC allograft), for the duration of severe neutropenia. The risk of resistance selection must be constantly assessed.

- **Antifungal prophylaxis :**

o **Anti-mould (posaconazole, voriconazole):** Recommended in patients at very high risk of invasive aspergillosis (induction AML/MDS, allograft patients with GVH).

o **Anti-Candida (fluconazole, micafungin):** Can be used if the main risk is candidiasis and not aspergillosis (e.g. autograft, certain phases of treatment in ALL).

- **Antiviral prophylaxis :**

o **Anti-HSV/VZV (aciclovir/valaciclovir) :** Systematic in HSV/VZV-positive patients undergoing intensive chemotherapy or HSC transplantation.

o Anti-CMV prophylaxis (letermovir) in certain CMV seropositive allograft patients at high risk of reactivation.

- **Anti-Pneumocystis *jirovecii* (PJP) prophylaxis :**

o **Cotrimoxazole (or alternatives):** Indicated during and after intensive immunosuppressive treatments (ALL, allograft, fludarabine, alemtuzumab, prolonged corticosteroid therapy).

Conclusion

Febrile neutropenia in patients with haematological malignancies represents a major clinical challenge due to the depth and duration of immunosuppression, exposing them to a high risk of bacterial, fungal and viral infections that are often severe and polymicrobial. Most of these patients are considered to be at high risk of complications, requiring hospitalisation and empirical broad-spectrum intravenous antibiotic therapy, often initial dual therapy and more liberal PGC coverage. Suspicion and early management of invasive fungal infections are particularly crucial. Anti-infective prophylaxis strategies (antibacterial, antifungal, antiviral, anti-PJP) and the use of G-CSF are essential components of overall management to reduce infectious morbidity and mortality in this highly vulnerable population. Close collaboration between haematologists, oncologists, infectious diseases specialists and microbiologists is essential.

References

1. Freifeld AG, Bow EJ, Sepkowitz KA, et al. Clinical practice guideline for the use of antimicrobial agents in neutropenic patients with cancer: 2010 update by the Infectious Diseases Society of America. Clin Infect Dis. 2011;52(4):e56-e93.
2. Baden LR, Swaminathan S, Angarone M, et al. Prevention and Treatment of Cancer-Related Infections, Version 2.2016, NCCN Clinical Practice Guidelines in Oncology. J Natl Compr Canc Netw. 2016;14(7):882-913.
3. Klastersky J, de Naurois J, Rolston K, et al. Management of febrile neutropaenia: ESMO Clinical Practice Guidelines. Ann Oncol. 2016;27(suppl 5):v111-v118.
4. Estey EH. Acute myeloid leukemia: 2019 update on risk-stratification and management. Am J Hematol. 2018;93(10):1267-1291.
5. Tomblyn M, Chiller T, Einsele H, et al. Guidelines for preventing infectious complications among hematopoietic cell transplantation recipients: a global perspective. Biol Blood Marrow Transplant. 2009;15(10):1143-1238.
6. Maertens J, Marchetti O, Herbrecht R, et al. European guidelines for antifungal management in leukemia and hematopoietic stem cell transplant recipients: summary of the ECIL 3-2009 Update. Bone Marrow Transplant. 2011;46(5):709-718.
7. Taplitz RA, Kennedy EB, Bow EJ, et al. Antimicrobial Prophylaxis for Adult Patients With Cancer-Related Immunosuppression: ASCO and IDSA Clinical Practice Guideline Update. J Clin Oncol. 2018;36(30):3043-3054.

Chapter 15: Central Venous Catheter Infections (CVI) in the Neutropenic Patient

Introduction

Central venous catheters (CVCs), whether tunnelled catheters, implantable chambers (ICPs) or peripherally inserted central catheters (PICC lines), are essential devices in the management of cancer patients. They are used to administer chemotherapy, transfusions, repeated blood sampling and parenteral nutrition [1]. However, they are also a major point of entry for micro-organisms and are a frequent cause of infection, particularly bacteraemia, in immunocompromised patients, particularly during periods of febrile neutropenia (NF) [2]. Early diagnosis of a catheter-associated infection (CAI), appropriate antibiotic therapy, sometimes including antibiotic "locks", and a judicious decision as to whether or not to remove the catheter are crucial to management. Rigorous preventive measures are also essential to minimise this risk [3]. This chapter details the diagnostic approach, therapeutic strategies, indications for CVC removal and preventive measures for CLI.

15.1 Definitions and epidemiology of catheter-related infections (CLI)

. *15.1.1* **Key definitions [2, 3] :**

o **Catheter colonisation:** Presence of micro-organisms on the catheter (e.g. quantitative culture of the catheter segment >15 CFU) without clinical signs of infection.

o **Infection of the insertion site or subcutaneous tunnel:** Inflammatory signs (erythema, induration, pain, purulent discharge) in an area <2 cm around the catheter port or along the subcutaneous path of the tunnelled catheter, without signs of associated bacteremia.

o **Catheter-Related Bacteremia/Fungemia (CRBF):** Isolate the same organism (same species and same antibiogram) in a peripheral blood culture AND in a blood culture taken from the CVC (or from a catheter segment sample), with clinical signs of infection, and without any other obvious infectious site.

■ An important criterion for BRLC is the **Differential Positivity Time (DTP)** of blood cultures: a positive result in blood cultures taken from the CVC occurring at least **2 hours before** that in peripheral blood cultures is strongly suggestive of a catheter origin of the bacteremia (if the bottles were incubated simultaneously and with an equivalent volume of blood).

- 15.1.2 Epidemiology and common pathogens :

o CLIs are a major cause of nosocomial infections and bacteraemia in cancer patients.

○ **Most common pathogens [2, 4] :**

■ **Gram-positive cocci:** *Staphylococcus epidermidis* and other coagulase-negative staphylococci (SCN) are the most common (often derived from skin flora). *Staphylococcus aureus* (MRSA or MSSA). Enterococci.

■ **Gram-negative bacilli**: Less common but often more serious (*Klebsiella spp., Enterobacter spp., Pseudomonas aeruginosa*, etc.).

■ **Yeasts:** *Candida spp.* (especially if parenteral nutrition or prolonged broad-spectrum antibiotic therapy).

○ Polymicrobial infections are possible.

○ Biofilm formation on the catheter: micro-organisms adhere to the catheter surface and produce a protective matrix, making them more difficult to eradicate with systemic antibiotics alone.

15.2 Diagnosis of Catheter-Related Infections

The diagnosis of CLI is based on a combination of clinical and microbiological evidence [2, 3, 5].

- **15.2.1 Evocative clinical signs :**

○ Fever, chills (especially if they occur during or shortly after a CVC infusion).

○ Local inflammatory signs at the CVC insertion site or along the tunnel (erythema, pain, induration, purulent discharge).

○ Catheter malfunction (difficulty infusing or sampling).

○ No other obvious infectious site to explain the fever.

- **15.2.2 Microbiological samples :**

○ **Paired blood cultures (systematic if CLI with systemic signs is suspected):**

■ At least one pair of blood cultures taken from **each CVC lumen** AND at least one pair of blood cultures taken from **peripheral venous**.

■ The time of sampling and the volume must be accurately recorded in order to calculate the DTP.

CVC port sampling: Swab if purulent discharge (for direct examination and culture).

○ **Catheter segment culture:** If the catheter is removed for suspected infection, send the distal tip (approximately 5 cm) and any intradermal segment to the laboratory for semi-quantitative (Maki method >15 CFU) or quantitative (sonication >100-1000 CFU) culture.

- 15.2.3 Interpretation of results and diagnostic criteria :

○ **BRLC confirmed if :**

■ Same micro-organism isolated from peripheral blood AND from the catheter (segment or blood culture from CVC).

■ AND DTP > 2 hours in favour of the CVC.
■ OR quantitative culture of the catheter segment significantly higher (>3-5 times) than that of the peripheral blood cultures (if lysis centrifugation method).
o A positive blood culture only on the CVC (without peripheral positivity) may indicate colonisation or an incipient infection limited to the catheter.
o The presence of SCN in a single blood culture (peripheral or CVC) is often interpreted as contamination, unless there are clear clinical signs of CLI or several blood cultures are positive for the same SCN.

15.3 Treatment of catheter-related infections

Management of CLI depends on the clinical severity, the type of catheter, the pathogen involved, and whether or not the catheter can be retained [2, 3, 5, 6]. An infectious diseases opinion is often required.

- **15.3.1 Systemic antibiotic therapy :**

o **Empirical initiation:** If CLB is suspected in a febrile neutropenic patient, initial empirical antibiotic therapy should cover the most likely pathogens, including PFMC. The addition of **vancomycin (or teicoplanin)** is therefore often justified as first-line therapy in this context (see Chapter 6.4).
o **Secondary adaptation:** Once the pathogen has been identified and its antibiogram obtained, antibiotic therapy should be adapted to a narrower, targeted spectrum.
o **Duration:**
■ If BRLC without complications (e.g. endocarditis, septic thrombophlebitis, osteomyelitis) and catheter removal: 7-14 days.
■ If catheter retention is attempted: 10-14 days of systemic antibiotic therapy, often supplemented by an antibiotic lock.
■ If infection with *S. aureus* or *Candida spp.*: often a minimum of 14 days, and catheter removal strongly recommended.
■ If complications arise (endocarditis, etc.): prolonged treatment (4-6 weeks or more).

• **15.3.2 Antibiotic Lock Therapy (ALT) :**

o **Principle:** Instillation of a high concentration antibiotic solution into the lumen of the colonised/infected catheter, left in place for several hours (generally 12-24h) between catheter uses. The aim is to eradicate the biofilm.
o **Indications :** Used as a complement to systemic antibiotic therapy with the aim of preserving a tunnelled catheter or CIP, in cases of uncomplicated CLI, with SCN or certain susceptible BGN, and in the absence of signs of infection of the tunnel or the lodge.
o **Molecules used :** Vancomycin, teicoplanin, gentamicin, ciprofloxacin,

ceftazidime, 70% ethanol, etc., often in combination with an anticoagulant (heparin, citrate) to prevent thrombosis. The choice depends on the germ.

- **Duration:** Usually 10-14 days.
- ALT is not indicated for *S. aureus*, *Pseudomonas aeruginosa*, or *Candida spp.* infections, where catheter removal is preferred.

• **15.3.3 Systemic antifungal treatment :**

- If catheter-related fungemia (mainly *Candida spp.*):

■ **Systematic and urgent catheter removal.**

■ Systemic antifungal treatment (echinocandin as first-line treatment, then fluconazole if sensitive strain) for at least 14 days after the first negative blood culture AND resolution of signs/symptoms.

■ Examination of the eye fundus to look for ocular localization.

15.4 Indications for central venous catheter removal

The decision to remove a CVC for CLI is crucial and depends on several factors [2, 3, 5, 6].

• **Systematic and Urgent Catheter Withdrawal Recommended if :**

- **Severe sepsis or septic shock.**
- **Persistent haemodynamic instability** despite appropriate antibiotic therapy.
- **Endocarditis or suppurative thrombophlebitis** (septic thrombosis of the vein where the catheter is located).
- ***Staphylococcus aureus* infection.**
- **Infection with *Pseudomonas aeruginosa* or other difficult-to-treat BGN.**
- **Fungemia (all species of *Candida spp*. or other fungi).**
- **Infection with atypical mycobacteria.**
- **Infection of the subcutaneous tunnel or the IPC lodge.**
- **Persistence of bacteremia/fungemia > 72 hours** despite appropriate antibiotic therapy and antibiotic lock (if attempted).
- **Impossible to administer effective systemic antibiotic therapy.**

• **Withdrawal to be discussed (Attempted preservation possible with ALT if long-term catheter and uncomplicated CLI):**

- Uncomplicated infection with Coagulase Negative Staphylococcus (CNS).
- Uncomplicated infection with certain susceptible Enterobacteriaceae, if the patient is stable and responds well to treatment.

• **If the catheter is removed:** If possible, do not replace it immediately at the same site. Wait for negative blood cultures and clinical resolution.

15.5 Prevention of Catheter-Related Infections

Prevention is the most effective strategy for reducing the incidence of CLI [2, 3, 7]. It is based on a set of measures ("bundles") to be applied rigorously:

- **Training for nursing staff:** Techniques for inserting, maintaining and aseptically handling CVCs.
- **Choice of catheter type and insertion site:**

o Choose the most suitable catheter with the fewest lumens required.

o Give preference to the subclavian vein in adults (less risk of infection than jugular or femoral), unless there are contraindications.

- **Rigorous asepsis during CVC insertion:**

o Maximum hand hygiene.

o Maximum barrier precautions (wide sterile drape, gown, mask, sterile gloves).

o Thorough skin disinfection with an alcoholic solution of chlorhexidine (>0.5%) or povidone iodine (allow sufficient drying time).

- **Maintenance and Aseptic Handling of the CVC :**

o Hand hygiene before handling.

o Disinfection of tips and injection sites before each use (e.g. with chlorhexidine alcohol solution or 70% alcohol swabs).

o Semi-permeable transparent sterile dressing (to be changed every 57 days or if soiled/unstuck) or opaque dressing (to be changed every 2-3 days). The use of chlorhexidine-impregnated dressings may reduce the risk in some patients.

o Limit the number of manipulations and connections.

o Change infusion lines as recommended (e.g. every 72-96 hours for continuous infusions, every 24 hours for lipids or blood).

- **Insertion Site Monitoring:** Daily inspection for signs of inflammation.
- **Catheter removal as soon as it is no longer essential.**
- **Use of Catheters Impregnated with Antiseptics/Antibiotics**

Can be discussed for patients at very high risk of CLI, but their routine use is not universally recommended because of the cost and the risk of resistance selection.

- **Prophylactic locks (e.g. taurolidine, citrate):** Their place in prophylaxis has yet to be defined and is reserved for specific situations.

Table 15.1: Risk stratification and additional measures

Level of Risk	Patient characteristics	Specific measures
Standard	Neutropenia <7 days	Basic Bundle
High	Neutropenia >7 days + mucositis grade >3	Silver-impregnated catheter + antibiotic lock
Very high	Previous CLI or BMR colonisation	Tunnelled catheter + prophylactic IV vancomycin

Conclusion

Central venous catheter-associated infections are a frequent and potentially serious complication in febrile neutropenic patients. Diagnosis is based on a high degree of clinical suspicion and rigorous microbiological sampling, in particular matched blood cultures with calculation of the differential time of positivity. Therapeutic management combines appropriate systemic antibiotic therapy and, in some cases, antibiotic locks, but catheter removal is often necessary, particularly for severe infections or infections with virulent germs such as *S. aureus* or *Candida spp*. The prevention of CLI, based on strict asepsis during catheter insertion and handling, as well as rigorous maintenance protocols, remains the cornerstone for reducing the incidence of these infections and improving the safety of patients with CVCs.

References

1. Bishop L, Dougherty L, Bodenham A, et al. Guidelines on the insertion and management of central venous access devices in adults. Int J Lab Hematol. 2007;29(4):261-278.

2. Mermel LA, Allon M, Bouza E, et al. Clinical practice guidelines for the diagnosis and management of intravascular catheter-related infection: 2009 Update by the Infectious Diseases Society of America. Clin Infect Dis. 2009;49(1):1-45.

3. O'Grady NP, Alexander M, Burns LA, et al. Guidelines for the Prevention of Intravascular Catheter-Related Infections, 2011. Clin Infect Dis. 2011;52(9):e162-e193.

4. Wisplinghoff H, Bischoff T, Tallent SM, et al. Nosocomial bloodstream infections in US hospitals: analysis of 24,179 cases from a prospective nationwide surveillance study. Clin Infect Dis. 2004;39(3):309-317.

5. Raad I, Hanna H, Maki D. Intravascular catheter-related infections: advances in diagnosis, prevention, and management. Lancet Infect Dis. 2007;7(10):645-657.

6. Freifeld AG, Bow EJ, Sepkowitz KA, et al. Clinical practice guideline for the use of antimicrobial agents in neutropenic patients with cancer: 2010 update by the Infectious Diseases Society of America. Clin Infect Dis. 2011;52(4):e56-e93.

7. French Society of Hospital Hygiene (SF2H). Recommendations for the prevention of infections associated with central vascular catheters.

Chapter 16: Impact of Bacterial Resistance on the Management of Febrile Neutropenia

Introduction

The emergence and increasing spread of multi-drug resistant (MDR) and highly antibiotic resistant (HAR) bacteria represent a major threat to global public health and a particularly critical challenge in the management of febrile neutropenic patients [1, 2]. Because of their immunosuppression and frequent exposure to antibiotics and the hospital environment, these patients are at high risk of infections with resistant germs, which are associated with increased morbidity, mortality, length of hospital stay and healthcare costs [3]. Knowledge of the main resistance mechanisms, appropriate antibiotic therapy strategies in the event of suspected or documented infection with BMR/BHRe, the importance of local epidemiology, and measures to prevent their spread are essential to optimise the management of febrile neutropenia in this worrying context [4].

16.1 Emergence and spread of Multi-resistant Bacteria (MRB) and Highly Resistant Bacteria (HRB)

- 16.1.1 Definitions :

○ **Multi-resistant bacteria (MRB):** Bacteria resistant to at least three different classes of antibiotics among those usually active on this species.

○ **Emerging Highly Antibiotic Resistant Bacteria (HARB) :** Category defined by the health authorities (e.g. Santé Publique France) including bacteria presenting resistance of particular concern for public health, such as Carbapenemase-producing Enterobacteriaceae (CPE) or Vancomycin-resistant *Enterococcus faecium* (VRE) [5]. Other international definitions exist (e.g. XDR - Extensively Drug-Resistant, PDR - Pandrug-Resistant).

- 16.1.2 Main BMR/BHRe of concern in cases of febrile neutropenia :

○ **Extended-spectrum beta-lactamase-producing Enterobacteriaceae (EBLSE) :**

■ *Escherichia coli* and *Klebsiella pneumoniae* are the most common.

■ Resistant to most penicillins and cephalosporins (including C3G/C4G).

■ Often associated with co-resistances (fluoroquinolones, aminosides, cotrimoxazole).

■ Carbapenems generally remain active, but their extensive use encourages the emergence of EPCs.

○ **Carbapenemase-producing Enterobacteriaceae (EPC):**

■ Ex: *Klebsiella pneumoniae* producing KPC (Klebsiella Pneumoniae Carbapenemase), NDM (New Delhi Metallo- beta-lactamase), OXA-48.

■ Resistant to most beta-lactams, including carbapenems.

■ Very limited treatment options, often combinations of antibiotics (e.g. ceftazidime-avibactam, meropenem-vaborbactam, imipenem-relebactam, cefiderocol, colistin, tigecycline, fosfomycin, certain aminoglycosides) [1, 6].

■ Associated with high mortality.

o **Resistant *Pseudomonas aeruginosa*:**

■ Can develop resistance to several classes (piperacillin-tazobactam, ceftazidime/cefepime, carbapenems, fluoroquinolones, aminoglycosides).

■ *P. aeruginosa*, which produces carbapenemases (metallo-beta lactamases in particular) or is multi-resistant (MDR-PA), is particularly difficult to treat.

o **Meticillin-resistant *Staphylococcus aureus* (MRSA):**

■ Resistant to all beta-lactams (except ceftaroline, ceftobiprole).

■ Treatment with glycopeptides (vancomycin, teicoplanin), linezolid, daptomycin, tigecycline, etc.

o **Vancomycin-resistant *Enterococcus faecium* (VRE):**

■ Growing problem, especially *E. faecium*.

■ Limited therapeutic options (linezolid, daptomycin, tigecycline, quinupristin-dalfopristin).

o Other BMR/BHRe: carbapenem-resistant *Acinetobacter baumannii*, *Stenotrophomonas maltophilia* (naturally resistant to many antibiotics).

Table 16.1: Main BMR/BHRe in the context of febrile neutropenia

Bacteria	Mechanisms of resistance	Therapeutic options	Mortality Associated
EBLSE (E. coli, K. pneumoniae)	BLSE (CTX-M, SHV, TEM)	Carbapenems Cefiderocol Ceftazidime-avibactam (if not EPC)	15-30%
EPC (KPC, NDM, OXA-48)	Carbapenemases	Ceftazidime-avibactam (KPC/OXA-48) Meropenem-vaborbactam Colistin + high-dose carbapenem	40-60%
Pseudomonas MDR	Porins + carbapenemases	Ceftolozane-tazobactam Cefiderocol Colistin + fosfomycin	35-50%
MRSA	MecA (PBP2a)	Vancomycin (Target: AUC/MIC >400) Daptomycin (6-8 mg/kg) Ceftaroline	20-40%
VRE (E. faecium)	VanA/VanB	Linezolid Daptomycin Tedizolid	25-45%
Acinetobacter MDR	OXA-23/40/58	Colistin + high-dose meropenem Eravacycline	50-70%

- 16.1.3 Factors favouring the emergence and spread of resistance:

o Massive and inappropriate use of antibiotics (in human and veterinary medicine).

o Antibiotic selection pressure in hospitals.

o Failure to comply with hygiene and cross-transmission prevention measures.

o International travel.

o Cancer patients, who are often hospitalised, receive repeated antibiotic treatment and wear invasive devices, are particularly exposed to the risk of acquiring and carrying BMR/BHRe.

16.2 Empirical Antibiotic Therapy Strategies for Suspected BMR/BHRe Infection

The choice of empirical antibiotic therapy must be adapted if a patient is known to be a carrier of a BMR/BHRe or if he/she presents high risk factors for infection by such germs [1, 3, 4, 6].

- **16.2.1 Identification of Patients at Risk of BMR/BHRe Infection :**

o **Previous colonisation or recent documented infection** with a specific BMR/BHRe.

o Recent or prolonged hospitalisation in a department/hospital with a high prevalence of BMR/BHRe.

o Recent or prolonged broad-spectrum antibiotic therapy (particularly carbapenems, fluoroquinolones, C3G).

- Recent travel to an area where BMR/BHRe are highly endemic.
- Patient in critical condition (severe sepsis, septic shock) where inadequate initial coverage would be fatal.

- **16.2.2 Adaptation of Empirical Antibiotic Therapy :**

- **If there is a risk of EBLSE infection :**

▪ A **carbapenem (meropenem, imipenem)** is often the empirical treatment of choice if the patient is severe or if the EBLSE is also resistant to other classes.

▪

▪ Piperacillin-tazobactam may be an option if the strain is known to be susceptible and the infection is not severe (debate over its efficacy for severe EBLSE infections).

- **If there is a risk of EPC infection (colonised patient or worrying local epidemiology) AND severe sepsis/septic shock:**

▪ A **combination of antibiotics** is often required, based on susceptibility data for local strains or the patient if known.

▪ Examples: Ceftazidime-avibactam, meropenem-vaborbactam, imipenem-relebactam, cefiderocol, or a combination including colistin, tigecycline, IV fosfomycin, or a high-dose aminoglycoside (if still active) [6, 7].

▪ **Urgent and essential infectious diseases opinion.**

- **If there is a risk of MDR *P. aeruginosa* infection:**

▪ The choice will depend on known resistance. Combination therapy is often required, which may include a "strong" carbapenem (if susceptible), a new beta-lactam/beta-lactamase inhibitor (e.g. ceftolozane-tazobactam, ceftazidime- avibactam), cefiderocol, colistin, or an aminoglycoside.

- **If there is a risk of MRSA infection (known colonisation, catheter infection, severe pneumonia in an epidemic context):**

▪ Add vancomycin, teicoplanin, linezolid or daptomycin to the empirical antibiotic therapy.

- **If there is a risk of VRE infection (known colonisation, local epidemiology):**

▪ Linezolid or daptomycin.

16.3 Importance of local ecology and antibiotic susceptibility testing data Knowledge of the local epidemiology of bacterial resistance is fundamental in guiding the choice of empirical antibiotic therapy.

- **Local data surveillance:** Every healthcare establishment should have up-to-date data on the main pathogens isolated from febrile neutropenic patients and their antibiotic susceptibility profiles. These data can be used to adapt local protocols for empirical antibiotic therapy.

- **Role of the Microbiology Laboratory :**

o Rapid identification of pathogens.

o Complete antibiotic susceptibility testing, including the search for specific resistance mechanisms (ESBL, carbapenemases).

o Rapid communication of critical results to clinicians.

o Assistance in interpreting results and choosing antibiotics.

- **Systematic screening for the carriage of BMR/BHRe :**

o Rectal (for EPC, EBLSE, VRE) or nasal (for MRSA) carriage screening can be carried out on admission or before high-risk chemotherapy in patients at risk (repeated hospitalisations, inter-institution transfers, travel to endemic areas). Knowledge of carriage guides empirical antibiotic therapy in cases of NF.

- **Antimicrobial Stewardship:**

Antibiotic stewardship programmes are essential to promote the judicious use of antibiotics, optimise treatment and limit selection pressure and the emergence of resistance [4]. This includes systematic re-evaluation of antibiotic therapy, de-escalation and adherence to recommended treatment durations.

16.4 Hygiene measures to prevent the spread of BMR/BHRe

Preventing the cross-transmission of BMR/BHRe in hospitals is a major public health issue [5, 8].

- **Standard hygiene precautions :**

o **Rigorous hand hygiene** (hydro-alcoholic friction or washing with soap and water) by all carers, before and after each contact with the patient or the patient's environment. This is the most important measure.

o Wear gloves if there is a risk of contact with biological fluids.

- **Complementary Contact Precautions (CCP):**

o Indicated for patients known to be carriers or infected with certain BMR/BHRe (e.g. MRSA, VRE, EPC, *C. difficile*).

o Single room if possible.

o Gowns and single-use gloves must be worn during treatment.

o Dedicated patient care equipment (blood pressure monitor, stethoscope).

o Reinforced hand hygiene.

- **Environmental hygiene :**

o Twice-daily cleaning and disinfection of surfaces and equipment in the patient's room, using appropriate products.

- **Cohorting:** Group together patients who are carriers of the same BMR/BHRe in the same sector, with dedicated staff if possible (in epidemic situations).

- **Information and education:** for patients, visitors and nursing staff on hygiene measures.

Conclusion

The impact of bacterial resistance on the management of febrile neutropenia is a growing concern and a daily challenge for clinicians. The emergence of BMR and especially BHRe such as EPC drastically limits therapeutic options and is associated with a poorer prognosis. A proactive strategy is essential, based on knowledge of the local epidemiology of resistance, identification of patients at risk of BMR/BHRe infection so that empirical antibiotic therapy can be adapted, judicious use of antibiotics (antibiotic governance), and rigorous application of hygiene measures to prevent their spread. Collaboration between oncologists/haematologists, infectious diseases specialists, microbiologists, pharmacists and hospital hygiene teams is more crucial than ever to tackle this threat and preserve the efficacy of our antibiotics for future generations of neutropenic patients. References

1. Tacconelli E, Carrara E, Savoldi A, et al. Discovery, research, and development of new antibiotics: the WHO priority list of antibioticresistant bacteria and tuberculosis. Lancet Infect Dis. 2018;18(3):318-327.

2. World Health Organization (WHO). Global antimicrobial resistance and use surveillance system (GLASS) report: 2021. Geneva: WHO; 2021.

3. Zilberberg MD, Shorr AF, Micek ST, et al. Epidemiology and outcomes of hospitalizations with complicated urinary tract infections in the United States, 2000-2009. Infect Control Hosp Epidemiol. 2013;34(10):1099- 1104.

4. Barlam TF, Cosgrove SE, Abbo LM, et al. Implementing an antibiotic stewardship program: guidelines by the Infectious Diseases Society of America and the Society for Healthcare Epidemiology of America. Clin Infect Dis. 2016;62(10):e51-e77.

5. Santé Publique France. Surveillance of emerging Highly Antibiotic Resistant Bacteria (HARB).

6. Karaiskos I, Giamarellou H. Multidrug-resistant Gram-negative bacterial infections: a new era of old and new antibiotics. Expert Rev Anti Infect Ther. 2014;12(1):81-100.

7. Timsit JF, Soubirou JL, Voiriot G, et al. Treatments for infections caused by carbapenem-resistant Gram-negative bacilli: a review. JAMA Intern Med. 2020;180(12):1632-1642.

8. Siegel JD, Rhinehart E, Jackson M, Chiarello L; Healthcare Infection Control Practices Advisory Committee. Management of multidrug-resistant organisms in healthcare settings, 2006.

Chapter 17: Research and Future Perspectives in the Management of Febrile Neutropenia

Introduction

The management of febrile neutropenia (NF) has progressed considerably in recent decades, leading to a significant improvement in the prognosis of cancer patients. However, major challenges remain, including the emergence of bacterial resistance, the difficulty of early diagnosis of specific infections, and the need to optimise the use of resources and support treatments. Scientific and clinical research is therefore intensely active in developing new diagnostic, therapeutic and preventive approaches [1, 2]. This chapter explores the most promising avenues of research, including new biomarkers, therapeutic innovations and the optimisation of support strategies, and highlights the crucial importance of scientific collaboration in meeting future challenges.

17.1 New biomarkers for early diagnosis of infections and risk stratification

Rapid identification of the cause of a fever in a neutropenic patient and precise stratification of the risk of complications are major challenges for individualised management. Research into new biomarkers is therefore a priority [3, 4].

- 17.1.1 Improvement of existing biomarkers :

○ **Procalcitonin (PCT):** Studies continue to evaluate its optimal role in distinguishing bacterial infections from other causes of fever, in guiding antibiotic de-escalation, and in predicting severity [4, 5]. Algorithms integrating PCT with other parameters are under development.

Ultrasensitive CRP (hs-CRP): Its usefulness in combination with other markers is being explored.

- **17.1.2 New Proteomic and Cytokine Biomarkers :**

○ **Cytokine/chemokine panels:** Analysis of specific cytokine (e.g. IL-6, IL-8, IL-10, TNF-a) or chemokine profiles could enable earlier identification of the type of infection (bacterial, fungal, viral) or the severity of sepsis [6].

○ **Pentraxin 3 (PTX3):** Acute phase protein produced locally at the site of inflammation, potentially more specific than CRP for infections.

○ **Neutrophil CD64 (nCD64)**: Expression of the CD64 receptor on the surface of neutrophils increases in the event of bacterial infection and could be an early marker of sepsis.

○ **Other markers of endothelial activation or host response** (e.g. Presepsin (sCD14-ST), suPAR (soluble urokinasetype plasminogen activator receptor)).

- **17.1.3 Metabolomic and transcriptomic biomarkers :**

○ Analysis of metabolomic (metabolites in blood or urine) or transcriptomic (gene expression in blood cells) profiles could reveal specific signatures associated with different types of infection or an increased risk of complications [7]. These 'omics' approaches are promising but require validation.

- **17.1.4 Improved fungal and viral biomarkers :**

○ Development of faster and more sensitive multiplex PCR tests for the detection of a wide range of fungal or viral pathogens directly from blood or other samples.

○ Improved standardisation and interpretation of the (1 ^3)-ß-D-Glucan and Galactomannan Antigen tests.

- 17.1.5 Data Integration and Artificial Intelligence (AI):

AI-based predictive models, integrating multiple clinical, biological and biomarker data, could enable more refined and personalised risk stratification, as well as aiding aetiological diagnosis [8].

17.2 New anti-infective therapeutic approaches

Faced with the growing threat of bacterial resistance, the development of new anti-infective strategies is an absolute priority.

- 17.2.1 New classes of antibiotics and new agents:

The pipeline of new antibiotics, although smaller than before, contains some promising molecules, particularly against multi-resistant BGN and EPC [9, 10]:

○ **New beta-lactamase inhibitor/beta-lactam combinations:** Ceftazidime-avibactam, meropenem-vaborbactam, imipenem-cilastatin-relebactam, ceftolozane-tazobactam (enhanced activity against MDR *P. aeruginosa*).

○ **Cefiderocol: a** siderophore cephalosporin with activity against many resistant BGN, including EPC and MDR *P. aeruginosa*, thanks to its "Trojan horse" entry mechanism. ○ **New tetracyclines (e.g. eravacycline, omadacycline) and aminoglycosides (e.g. plazomicin)** with improved activity against certain resistant germs.

○ Molecules targeting new bacterial pathways.

- **17.2.2 Phage therapy :**

Use of bacteriophages (viruses that specifically infect and lyse bacteria) as an alternative or complement to antibiotics, particularly for BMR/BHRe infections. This is a fast-growing area of research, but there are still challenges in terms of regulation, production and clinical trials [11].

- **17.2.3 Immunomodulation strategies and adjuvant therapies :**

○ **Modulation of the host response:** Explore molecules capable of reinforcing the patient's immune defences (apart from G-CSF) or modulating the deleterious inflammatory response of sepsis, without compromising anti-tumour activity.

○ **Anti-bacterial or anti-toxin monoclonal antibodies:** In development to specifically target certain pathogens or their virulence factors.

○ **Antimicrobial peptides.**

○ **Probiotics and modulation of the microbiota:** Potential role in preventing infections by competing with pathogens or restoring a protective microbiota (see also section 17.3).

- **17.2.4 New Antifungals and Antivirals :**

○ Development of new classes of antifungal agents (e.g. DHODH inhibitors such as olorofim for rare moulds, new azoles).

○ Research into broader-spectrum antivirals or those targeting emerging viruses.

17.3 Optimising the use of G-CSF and prophylaxis

Although G-CSF and anti-infective prophylaxis are valuable tools, their use must be optimised to maximise their benefit and minimise their inconvenience.

- **17.3.1 More targeted use of G-CSF :**

○ Refine the indications for primary prophylaxis in intermediate-risk regimens using more effective individual risk scores incorporating patient-specific factors (genetics, biomarkers).

○ Find the optimal administration regimen (dose, duration, type of G-CSF) for each clinical situation.

○ Better define the role of biosimilar G-CSFs.

- **17.3.2 Personalised anti-infective prophylaxis strategies :**

○ **Antibacterial prophylaxis:** Develop strategies to limit the impact on the microbiota and the emergence of resistance (e.g. intermittent prophylaxis, targeted decolonisation, use of narrower spectrum molecules if possible). The role of non-absorbable antibiotics is being explored.

○ **Antifungal prophylaxis:** better identification of patients who really benefit from antifungal prophylaxis, potentially using risk biomarkers.

○ **Modulation of the microbiota as a prophylactic strategy:** Use of specific probiotics or prebiotics to maintain a healthy intestinal flora and prevent bacterial/fungal translocation. Transplantation of faecal microbiota is being studied in the context of severe dysbiosis or recurrent *C. difficile* infection, but its role in the primary prophylaxis of NF remains to be defined [12].

- **17.3.3 Optimisation of vaccination programmes :**
  - Develop more immunogenic vaccines for immunocompromised patients.
  - Better define the optimal timing of vaccinations in relation to chemotherapy cycles or immunosuppression.
  - Strategies to improve vaccination coverage in cancer patients and their families.

17.4 Importance of Collaborative Studies and Registries

To advance research and improve the management of NF, large-scale collaboration is essential.

- **Multicentre Randomised Clinical Trials :**
  - Necessary to assess the efficacy and safety of new biomarkers, new therapeutic approaches (antibiotics, phagotherapy, immunomodulators) and optimised prophylaxis strategies.
  - Often difficult to conduct for specific populations or rare infections without broad collaboration.
- **Registries and prospective cohorts :**
  - Collect "real-life" data on large numbers of patients, study the epidemiology of NF and resistance, identify risk and prognostic factors, and assess the impact of different management strategies.
  - Crucial for monitoring BMR/BHRe and adapting local recommendations.
- **National and international research networks:**
  - Facilitate data sharing, harmonisation of protocols, and the conduct of collaborative studies.
  - Examples: Oncology cooperative groups (EORTC, etc.), infection surveillance networks (e.g. ECIL in Europe for infections in leukaemia patients).
- **Data sharing and Open Science :**

Initiatives to facilitate the sharing of research data (while respecting confidentiality) can accelerate discoveries and the validation of new approaches.

Conclusion

The management of febrile neutropenia is a constantly evolving field, driven by persistent challenges and advances in research. The development of new biomarkers for earlier diagnosis and more accurate risk stratification, the arrival of new classes of antibiotics and innovative therapeutic approaches such as phage therapy, and the optimisation of prevention and support strategies all offer promising prospects for further improving patient prognosis. The integration of artificial intelligence could also transform our approach. However, these advances cannot be achieved without a sustained effort in basic and clinical research, and without close collaboration between researchers, clinicians, the pharmaceutical industry and regulatory agencies. Collaborative studies and registries will play a key role in generating the necessary evidence and rapidly translating discoveries into concrete improvements for cancer patients facing the risk of febrile neutropenia.

References

1. Gudiol C, Akova M, Calandra T, et al. Management of febrile neutropenia in cancer patients: 2023 EORTC-IDSA-MSG-ESCMID guidelines. Lancet Oncol. 2023;

2. World Health Organization (WHO). Antimicrobial resistance: global report on surveillance. Geneva: WHO; 2014

3. Lisy K, Peters M, Schofield P, Jefford M. Identifying unmet needs of haematology cancer survivors: A systematic review. Support Care Cancer. 2018;26(6):1763-1775.

4. Garnacho-Montero J, Garcia-Garmendia JL, Barrero-Almodovar A, et al. Impact of adequate empirical antibiotic therapy on the outcome of patients admitted to the intensive care unit with sepsis. Crit Care Med. 2003;31(12):2742-2751.

5. Schuetz P, Beishuizen A, Broyles M, et al. Procalcitonin (PCT)-guided antibiotic stewardship: an international multidisciplinary consensus on optimized clinical use. Clin Chem Lab Med. 2017;55(10):1427-1439.

6. Pierrakos C, Vincent JL. Sepsis biomarkers: a review. Crit Care. 2010;14(1):R15.

7. McComb S, Thwaites R, Tregoning JS. Metabolomics of infection: a review. Philos Trans R Soc Lond B Biol Sci. 2019;374(1772):20180262.

8. Wiens J, Saria S, Sendak M, et al. Do P, et al. Do we need a new "omics" for AI in medicine? Nat Med. 2019;25(6):877-879.

9. Theuretzbacher U, Bush K, Harbarth S, et al. Critical new antibiotics are failing to address the threat of antibiotic-resistant bacteria. Lancet Infect Dis. 2020;20(6):e130-e141.

10. Bassetti M, Welte T, Wunderink RG. New antibiotics for ventilator-associated pneumonia. Curr Opin Crit Care. 2016;22(5):470-480.

11 Kortright KE, Chan BK, Koff JL, Turner PE. Phage Therapy: A Renewed Approach to Combat Antibiotic-Resistant Bacteria. Cell Host Microbe. 2019;25(2):219-232.

12 Van Nood E, Vrieze A, Nieuwdorp M, et al. Duodenal infusion of donor feces for recurrent Clostridium difficile. N Engl J Med. 2013;368(5):407-415.

General conclusion

Febrile Neutropenia, a Constant Challenge in Search of Continuous Optimisation

At the end of this book dedicated to febrile neutropenia (NF) in adult cancer patients, it is clear that this complication, although frequent and well studied, remains a major challenge and an unavoidable medical emergency in oncology and haematology. Its management has a direct impact on patient safety, the ability to deliver cancer treatment at the required dose and intensity, and ultimately on overall prognosis.

The aim of this handbook is to provide healthcare professionals with a comprehensive, practical and up-to-date overview of knowledge and strategies relating to NF. We have explored in detail the pathophysiology of neutropenia and the risk of infection, highlighting how neutrophil failure, coupled with impaired mucosal barriers, creates a breeding ground for serious infections. Mastery of the precise definitions and risk factors for the onset of NF, as well as factors predictive of complications, is the first step towards individualised management.

We stressed **the urgency of the initial clinical and paraclinical assessment**, with the need for a targeted history, a meticulous clinical examination (paying particular attention to "silent" sites), and rapid and relevant microbiological sampling before any antibiotic therapy. **Risk stratification**, in particular using validated scores such as the MASCC, is crucial in guiding the therapeutic decision: outpatient management with oral antibiotic therapy for low-risk patients meeting strict criteria, or hospitalisation with broad-spectrum intravenous antibiotic therapy for high-risk patients.

The "golden hour" concept for initiating empirical antibiotic therapy has been

reaffirmed as a quality of care standard, aimed at reducing morbidity and mortality. The choice of antibiotic molecules, detailed according to risk, local epidemiology and patient characteristics, should aim for optimal coverage of the most likely pathogens, while limiting the inappropriate use of very broad-spectrum agents or glycopeptides. **Systematic reassessment at H48-H72** is a key stage in adapting treatment, considering de-escalation or, on the contrary, intensifying management in the event of non-response, bearing in mind the possibility of fungal or viral infections.

Prevention of NF, through the judicious use of granulocyte growth factors (G-CSF) as primary or secondary prophylaxis, and through targeted anti-infective prophylaxis strategies in very high-risk patients, is an essential part of improving the tolerability of anti-cancer treatments. The specificities of NF in elderly patients or in the context of haematological malignancies, as well as the management of catheter-related infections, underlined the need for an approach tailored to each situation.

Finally, we addressed the growing challenge of **bacterial resistance**, which threatens the effectiveness of our antibiotics and calls for constant vigilance, rigorous antibiotic governance and strict compliance with hygiene measures. The outlook for the future, with the development of new biomarkers, new therapeutic approaches and the optimisation of existing strategies, opens up promising avenues, but also highlights the crucial importance of clinical research and collaborative studies.

In conclusion, the management of febrile neutropenia is a dynamic process that requires up-to-date knowledge, sharp clinical judgement, excellent coordination between the various healthcare professionals (oncologists, haematologists, infectiologists, emergency physicians, pharmacists, nurses), and clear communication with the patient. We hope that this book will be a valuable resource for all healthcare professionals, helping them to navigate the management of this oncological emergency with confidence and skill, with the constant aim of improving the safety, quality of life and prognosis of the patients they support in their fight against cancer. The quest for increasingly optimised management of febrile neutropenia is an ongoing commitment to our patients.

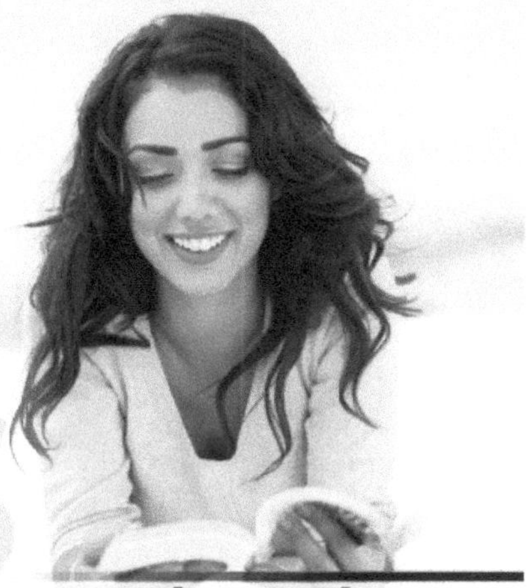

Kolibri 360 GmbH
Ferdinand-Jühlke-Straße 7
99095 Erfurt, Deutschland
produktsicherheit@kolibri360.de

Druck:
CPI Druckdienstleistungen GmbH
im Auftrag der
Kolibri 360 GmbH
Ferdinand-Jühlke-Str. 7
99095 Erfurt